Organizing for Independent Nursing Practice

Organizing for Independent Nursing Practice

Edited by

ADA K. JACOX, R.N., Ph.D.

Associate Dean for Research and Doctoral Program Development, University of Colorado Medical Center, Denver, Colorado

CATHERINE M. NORRIS, R.N., Ed.D.

Co-Project Director, Organization for the Practice of Psychiatric Nursing Conference, The University of Iowa, College of Nursing, Iowa City, Iowa

ACC Appleton-Century-Crofts/New York

Library of Congress Cataloging in Publication Data
Main entry under title:

Organizing for independent nursing practice.

Includes bibliographical references and index.
1. Nursing—Practice—Congresses. 2. Nurse practitioners—Congresses. I. Jacox, Ada K. II. Norris, Catherine M.
RT86.7.073 610.73 77-2188
ISBN 0-8385-7522-6

79 80 81 / 10 9 8 7 6 5 4 3 2

Prentice-Hall International, Inc., London
Prentice-Hall of Australia, Pty. Ltd., Sydney
Prentice-Hall of India Private Limited, New Delhi
Prentice-Hall of Japan, Inc., Tokyo
Prentice-Hall of Southeast Asia (Pte.) Ltd., Singapore
Whitehall Books Ltd., Wellington, New Zealand

PRINTED IN THE UNITED STATES OF AMERICA

CONTRIBUTORS

Patty Brandner, R.N., M.S.
Mental Health Nurse Therapist, Counseling Associates, Dallas, Texas

Kathleen C. Brown, R.N., M.S.
Family Nurse Practitioner, Community Health Nursing, School of Public Health & Tropical Medicine, Tulane University, New Orleans, Louisiana

Evelyn M. Chapman, R.N., M.A.
Family Nurse Practitioner, Big Piney, Wyoming

Marvin A. Fish
Attorney, Slavitt, Fish and Cowan, Newark, New Jersey

Loretta C. Ford, R.N., Ed.D.
Dean, School of Nursing, University of Rochester, Rochester, New York

Maddy Gerrish, R.N., Ph.D.
Owner/Clinical Director, Expansion, Inc., Bedford, Massachusetts

Mary Gray, R.N., M.N.Sc.
Family Nurse Practitioner, Director of Nurse Practitioner Training Program, College of Nursing, University of Arkansas for Medical Science, Little Rock, Arkansas

Mary Alice Hauser, R.N., M.A.
Mental Health Nurse, Iowa Veterans' Home, Marshalltown, Iowa

Marian Havlovic, R.N., M.S., C.A.N.A.-I.
Psychiatric Nurse, Private Practice, Chicago, Illinois

Karlene Kerfoot, R.N., M.A.
Nurse Practitioner, Lynn County Psychiatric Clinic, Cedar Rapids, Iowa

Elaine I. Nielsen, R.N.
Private Practice, Beresford, South Dakota

Lawrence I. Subrin, C.P.A.
Private Practice, Tucson, Arizona

Lynn Theuer, R.N., M.S.
Consultant, Nurse Psychotherapist, Officer and Stockholder, Nursing Consultation, Inc., Winona, Minnesota

Margaret Wacker, R.N., M.S., M.A.
Family Therapist, Private Practice, Dix Hills, New York

Carolyn V. Whitaker, R.N., M.S.N.
Family Nurse Practitioner, Red Boiling Springs, Tennessee

Anne Zimmerman, R.N.
President American Nurses' Association

Participants

Sarah Ellen Archer, R.N., Dr. P.H.
Community Nurse Practitioner, Nursing Dynamics Corp., Mill Valley, California

Maxine Bardach, R.N., M.A.
Psychotherapist, Private Practice, Northfield, Illinois

Patty Brandner, R.N., M.S.
Mental Health Nurse Therapist, Counseling Associates, Dallas, Texas

Kathleen C. Brown, R.N., M.S.
Family Nurse Practitioner, Community Health Nursing, School of Public Health & Tropical Medicine, Tulane University, New Orleans, Louisianna

Evelyn M. Chapman, R.N., M.A.
Family Nurse Practitioner, Big Piney, Wyoming

Jay Croley, R.N., M.A.
Gestalt Therapist, Private Practice, Albuquerque, New Mexico

Lorene Fischer, R.N., M.S.
Professor of Nursing, Director, Psychiatric-Mental Health Nursing Program, School of Nursing, Wayne State University, Detroit, Michigan

Sharon Gedan, R.N., M.S.
Group and Individual Psychotherapist, Honolulu, Hawaii

Maddy Gerrish, R.N., Ph.D.
Owner/Clinical Director, Expansion, Inc., Bedford, Massachusetts

Mary Gray, R.N., M.N. Sc.
Family Nurse Practitioner, Director of Nurse Practitioner Training Program, College of Nursing, University of Arkansas for Medical Science, Little Rock, Arkansas

Jocelyn A. Greenidge, R.N., M.A.
Community Nurse Practitioners, New York, New York

Leanne Halfman, R.N., M.S., S.N.P.
School Nurse Practitioner, Gary Community School Corporation, Gary, Indiana

Sister Carolita Hart, R.N., M.A.
Family Nurse Practitioner, North West Family Health Center, Salt Lake City, Utah

Mary Alice Hauser, R.N., M.A.
Mental Health Nurse, Iowa Veterans' Home, Marshalltown, Iowa

Marian Havlovic, R.N., M.S., C.A.N.A.-I
Psychiatric Nurse, Private Practice, Chicago, Illinois

Gertrude Isaacs, R.N., D. N.Sc.
Executive Director, Frontier Nursing Service, Hyden, Kentucky

Nancy Keller, R.N., Ph.D.
Partner, Nursing Care and Consultation, Ltd., Tucson, Arizona

Karlene Kerfoot, R.N., M.A.
Nurse Practitioner, Lynn County Psychiatric Clinic, Cedar Rapids, Iowa

Lucille Kinlein, R.N., M.S.N.E.
Independent Generalist Nurse, Hyattsville, Maryland

Mary Ann Lewis, R.N., M.A.
Director, Primex Project, Assistant Professor of Nursing and Medicine Health Science U.C.L.A., Los Angeles, California

Ingeborg Mauksch, R.N., Ph.D., F.A.A.N.
Professor and Family Nurse Clinician, School of Nursing, Vanderbilt University, Nashville, Tennessee

Nancy Milio, R.N., Ph.D.
Associate Dean and Professor, University of North Carolina, Chapel Hill, North Carolina

Elaine I. Nielsen, R.N.
Private Practice, Beresford, South Dakota

Janelle Smith Ramsburg, R.N., M.S.W.
Private Practice, Kansas City, Missouri

Janice E. Ruffin, R.N., M.S.
Director of Nursing, Connecticut Mental Health Center, Associate Professor, Yale University, School of Nursing, New Haven, Connecticut

Ada Shannon, R.N., M.A.
Pediatric Nurse Practitioner, San Jose, California

Nancy C. Talley, R.N., M.N.
Director of Ambulatory Care, St. Joseph's Hospital, Mental Health Center, Tampa, Florida

Lynn Theuer, R.N., M.S.
Consultant, Nurse Psychotherapist, Officer and Stockholder, Nursing Consultation, Inc., Winona, Minnesota

Sally Tripp, R.N., M.A.
Director, Nurse Practitioner Project, Division of Nursing, School of Health Sciences, University of Massachusetts, Amherst, Massachusetts

Josephine Vander Meer, R.N., Ph.D.
Director of Associate Degree Nursing Program, University of Albuquerque, Albuquerque, New Mexico

Margaret Wacker, R.N., M.S., M.A.
Family Therapist, Private Practice, Dix Hills, New York

Carolyn V. Whitaker, R.N., M.S.N.
Family Nurse Practitioner, Red Boiling Springs, Tennessee

Carolyn Williams, R.N., Ph.D.
Associate Professor, School of Nursing, University of North Carolina, Chapel Hill, North Carolina

Virginia Williams, R.N., M.A.
Private Practice, Family Nursing McHenry, Illinois

Advisory Committee for Conference

Evelyn Barritt, R.N., Ph.D.
Dean, College of Nursing, University of Iowa, Iowa City, Iowa

Elizabeth Carter, R.N., M.S.
Chairperson, Executive Committee of the Council of Psychiatric/Mental Health Nurses, A.N.A.; Assistant Professor, School of Nursing, Faculty of Medicine of Columbia University, New York, New York

Helen Grace, R.N., Ph.D.
Associate Dean for Graduate Study, School of Nursing, University of Illinois, Chicago, Illinois

Ada K. Jacox, R.N., Ph.D.
Associate Dean for Research and Doctoral Program, Development, School of Nursing, University of Colorado, Denver, Colorado

Catherine M. Norris, R.N., Ed.D.
Nursing Consultant, Tucson, Arizona

Representatives of Federal Agencies

M. Leah Gorman, R.N., Ed.D.
Chief, Graduate Education Section, Psychiatric Nursing Education Branch, Division of Manpower and Training Programs, National Institute of Mental Health, Washington, D.C.

Thomas Phillips, R.N., Ph.D.
Consultant, Nursing Research & Education Advisory Committee, Nursing Research Branch, Division of Nursing, Bureau of Health Manpower-Education, Department of Health, Education and Welfare, Washington, D.C.

Contents

Foreword

During many of my recent contacts with nurses, consumers, and newspaper and TV reporters over the country, the question of independent practice by nurse practitioners has inevitably come up. What is independent nursing practice, they ask. Who are nurse practitioners and how do they differ from just nurses? What do they do; where are they working? How many are there? And where and how does one learn to become an independent nurse practitioner? And so on.

Though the title, role, and qualifications of the "nurse practitioner" are still evolving and the advice of "go thou and do likewise" should prudently be offered to those contemplating practicing independently, this book–the proceedings of a special conference–offers a compilation of pioneering experiences described frankly by nurse practitioners themselves. It offers some wise advice, raises many telling questions, and deals with a myriad of critical issues, among them the important factors of qualifications, payment, support, and research.

Fee-for-service practice through individual contracts between nurses and patients, and in increasing instances through reimbursement by third-party payers, has been the economic base of private duty nursing in this country for years. Thus, while the idea of direct payment to a nurse for her services is not new, the nurse's being engaged in the independent practice of nursing is. And she is becoming known as a nurse practitioner whose role and function are described in various ways in this book.

This conference may be among the first to have been held to discuss organizing for independent nursing practice, but it certainly will not be the last. This book presents a great deal of material written in an interesting and often provocative style. I believe it merits the serious attention of nurses, consumers, physicians, and others who are concerned with nursing strategies and their impact on whatever national health policy emerges.

ANNE ZIMMERMAN, R.N.
President, American Nurses' Association

Introduction

In 1972 we began considering what means might be used to convene a group of nurse practitioners who were trying in various ways to practice nursing independently. We knew nurses who were "hanging out their shingles," and we read about and heard about many more. With some of them we discussed the problems they encountered, such as determining what services they would provide, learning to work their way through legal and business complexities, deciding what kinds of relationships with other professionals were appropriate, and so forth. What we heard repeatedly was how difficult it was to work through these problems alone and how eager these independent nurses were to know how others were dealing with similar problems. We thought that a small conference at which nurses who were in independent practice could share their experiences, knowledge, suggestions, and ideas would be a way to begin. In 1974, under the auspices of the College of Nursing at the University of Iowa, we wrote a proposal and went looking for financial support to implement our idea. In June of 1975 we were notified that the Psychiatric Nursing Education Branch of the National Institute of Mental Health had approved a grant (2T01 MH07600–14) to support a 2-day conference of nurse practitioners who were trying alternative practice arrangements.

This book is a report of that conference. It includes reports on issues and problems dealt with in small group meetings, papers presented by resource people, and excerpts of large group discussions. Participants were invited to prepare papers for the conference. A few did this, and a few brought copies of papers they had presented at other meetings. Several of these are included. Excerpts from other data collected from the participants before the conference are included to amplify the conference proceedings. The participants' evaluations of the conference are summarized.

The problems and issues on which the conference focused were dealt with to varying degrees of depth, and they aroused varying degrees of interest. The 2-day span of the conference did not permit exploration in great depth, although the many issues and problems identified provide some idea of the scope of the work to be done in the nurse practitioner movement. This report reflects the unevenness of emphasis and the varying thoroughness with which the issues were treated.

The report is organized into two sections. The first section includes papers presented at the conference, discussions following them, and reports of some of the small group sessions. The second section consists of five chapters, each of which is a composite of parts of several group discussions. We tried to organize the chapters in this section according to the major issues discussed by the participants in the several groups. Since many of the issues are interrelated, there is some overlap of content in the chapters.

Throughout the discussions, long descriptions of practice emerged. Where possible, the discussions relating to the practice of each nurse were pulled out and synthesized into a single description. Some of these are integrated into the various chapters where they seem to fit best, and a few descriptions are included in the Appendices. These detailed descriptions provide a rich source of data regarding the various issues involved in the nurse practitioner movement. They serve well to illustrate many of the ideas and problems discussed by the participants. In addition to the descriptions of practice, a copy of the program and a profile of the participants are included in the Appendices.

In preparing the report we tried to impose some organization on the material without misrepresenting the participants' ideas. Where possible, we identified each contributor in a discussion and sent the transcripts of these comments to the participants for validation of accuracy. Obviously, selectivity was involved in the choice of material to be included. We tried to include as many differing opinions on each issue as were expressed at the conference. Also, because this is a report, we documented the polarity of positions and feelings about the various issues, even though in places they seem over optimistic or very pessimistic. In a sense, the report is a summary of the experiences, ideas, and opinions of the conferees as observed and reported by us. In instances where reference was made to previous publications (eg, a research report or an analysis of the practitioner movement by another person), we went to those sources that were referenced in an attempt to fill in the details in the conference report.

There were some surprises in what emerged in the discussions. For example, we had a session identified as a policy session, in which we anticipated a discussion of establishing policy within a practice. However, the members of the group chose to focus on national policy, and Chapter 9, which is based largely on that discussion, makes a significant contribution to the examination of national policy issues. We had not anticipated a session on definitions of nursing, but this theme emerged repeatedly in both the small and large group discussions; Chapter 8 summarizes these discussions. While we had intended that discussion of the training of nurse practitioners be included, none of the groups really dealt with that issue.

For the purposes of the conference, it appears that there are two major groups of independent nurse practitioners. There are those who work for an agency or a physician but who carry their own client/patient load for whom they are responsible and accountable as primary caretakers. Then there are those who are in private practice alone, in partnership, or in corporations. Those in private practice have business, legal, public relations, and other concerns that employees do not have.

Some clarification of how we catagorized the conferees and how this relates to labels used by others might be useful here. Nonnurses and federal policy-making groups tend to use the terms physician's assistant and nurse practitioner together to designate those providing primary care and treatment under the supervision or written policies of a physician. Within nursing, the term nurse practitioner does not mean physician's assistant, although some of the functions of the nurse practitioner admittedly overlap those of the physician's assistant. Most nurses would agree that health care functions, advocacy functions, comfort functions, and counseling functions, at the minimum, are independent functions that the nurse is duly licensed to perform without medical input or supervision and that physician's assistants are neither prepared to perform nor licensed to perform. Beyond this, there are several terms used within nursing to identify this worker. Despite attempts within organized nursing to clarify the various kinds of nurses,* there is still a great deal of confusion within the profession about the differences among nurse practitioners, advanced practitioners,† nurse clinicians, clinical nurse specialists, and independent nurse practitioners.‡

Differences among these categories of nurses are viewed by some as involving level of skill and by others as involving scope of practice and variety of therapies offered. Still others focus on degree of knowledge and achievement of specified levels of education. To some nurses the degree of accountability, responsibility, and authority for an assigned case load of clients or patients is the determinant of an expanded nursing practice. To a large group of nurses the collaborative or supervisory relationship with a physician is the essence of the nurse's practice in an expanded role. And at least a few nurses firmly believe that the one word nurse says it all.

Many nurses are willing to accept a variety of terms as long as the terms are defined. But a great deal of concern has been expressed by a vocal majority that the public will be further confused about who is who in health care. They fear the kind of loss of identity the registered nurse suffered after World War II when we introduced nursing aides, nursing assistants, vocational nurses, licensed practical nurses, ward managers, and the like. For the purposes of this project, we used two terms to describe the participants. All participants in practice met the criteria of being independent nurse practitioners. That is, they all carried a case load of patients or clients whom they

**American Nurses' Association: Statement Clarifying Nurses' Roles. Congress for Nursing Practice, 1975*

†American Nurses' Association: Position Paper on Specialist Certification in Psychiatric Mental-Health Nursing. Council of Advanced Practitioners in Psychiatric Mental Health Nursing

‡American Nurses' Association: Statement on Third Party Payments for Services of Independent Nurse Practitioners. Commission on Economic and General Welfare, 1975

saw on a regular basis. They all carried out primary care activities and were accountable for the work they did with these clients/patients. This can involve working without a physician, working for a physician, working under medical policy or medical supervision, collaborating with a physician, being in joint practice with a physician, or employing physician consultants. The second group, private nurse practitioners, included those who in addition to being independent nurse practitioners were also in private practice as opposed to being an employee of a physician or a health care agency. Participants were categorized in this manner because the issues and problems involved with being in independent nursing practice as a salaried employee are different in many respects from those encountered by the self-employed nurse who sets up her own office and practices as a private practitioner of nursing.

The Advisory Committee for the conference did the work of planning and contributed greatly to the selection of participants. Members of the Advisory Committee were Evelyn R. Barritt, Dean of the College of Nursing, University of Iowa; Rosemary McKeighen, Director of the Psychiatric Mental Health Nursing Graduate Program, College of Nursing, University of Iowa; Elizabeth Carter, Chairperson of the Executive Committee of the Council of Advanced Practitioners in Psychiatric–Mental Health Nursing, American Nurses' Association; and Helen Grace, Associate Dean for Graduate Education in Nursing, School of Nursing, University of Illinois. The project's directors are grateful for the assistance of this group, both before and during the conference.

We wish to express our appreciation to M. Leah Gorman, Chief of the Graduate Education Section, Psychiatric Nursing Education Branch, National Institute of Mental Health, for her valuable advice and support of our efforts.

We would like to acknowledge the help of Kathleen Buckwalter, Dorothy Douglas, Ruth Ryan, and Mary Stewart, who assisted during the conference by recording the sessions. We also want to thank Shelley Etzel, Nancy Ristvedt, and Marge Landuyt for their cheerfulness and patience in taking protocols off tapes, typing several drafts of the report, and coping with all the unprogrammed events related to the conference.

We salute the participants themselves, who as pioneers are out there taking the risks and paving one route to the professional practice of nursing.

ADA K. JACOX
CATHERINE M. NORRIS
June, 1976

SECTION I

NURSING PRACTICE

CHAPTER 1

The Nurse Practitioner Conference

One of the most critical problems facing nursing today is the question of where the professional nurse can practice nursing. That we are now educating nurses competent to practice on a professional level is a comparatively recent development. Their numbers in nursing practice have been very small, because most of them have, up to this time, been recruited to work in universities. But now there are growing numbers of these nurses who want to practice professionally; that is, they want to fill critical gaps in health care that they are eminently equipped and qualified to fill. They want to be responsible and accountable for their own patients or, as they say, their own "patient care load." They want to control their own practice, to provide primary care and have primary therapeutic responsibility in their areas of expertise. They want to be paid adequately and directly for the services they provide. They want a voice in health care legislation, recognition at all levels of government of the contribution professional nursing can make, and support for nursing built into new legislation in the same way it is built in for other professions. These nurses are competent in the business and economic aspects of professional practice.

As women, professional nurses want to overcome the stereotypes involved in being both female and nurse: dependent female, mother surrogate, intellectual inferior. An end to these and myriad other stereotypes is required for the establishment of colleague relationships with other health professionals that allow cooperation and collaboration toward the end of improving health care.

Hospitals are not organized to accommodate this model of nursing. Although community clinics and public health nursing agencies evolved using the hospital model of practice, they do permit some of the criteria required by professional nurses to be met, at least in a limited way. Nursing education in general has been agency-oriented and has not provided the training or experience that would encourage nurses to develop their own nontraditional, nonmedical model of practice or to adopt the private practice model of the physician and other health professionals. Educational programs generally have not prepared nurses emotionally, intellectually, or practically to function on a colleague basis with other professionals, nor have they provided nurses the preparation necessary to enable them to move skillfully about in the various social and governmental strata of the community, including the health care system. Graduating nurses are usually politically naive. Educational programs have instilled little commitment for nurses to pressure actively for the freedom to perform those services they are uniquely prepared to provide for the people.

It has been left to a relatively small group of pioneers to explore new approaches: to work out partnerships with other professionals; to set up private practices, corporate clinics, community nursing services of various kinds; to organize contract services using a variety of treatment modalities, consultative activities, survey or screening procedures, and teaching services. The complexities of the legal, economic, business, and professional relationships, as well as public response, have made unsalaried arrangements for practice extremely difficult and often short-lived for some of these pioneers. But the number of successes appears to be increasing.

It is too early to say whether nursing practices in collaborative, independent, and private practitioner roles are viable options for professional nurses. There are forces within the profession and outside of it that may give impetus to what is yet a small, often controversial movement, and there are other forces that would suppress and discourage it.

PLANNING THE CONFERENCE

The general purpose of the project was to make a limited survey of the nurse practitioner movement in the area of psychiatric nursing by utilizing the conference method. The objectives of the project as submitted on the proposal were too ambitious for a 2-day working conference. They are included here as a matter of record and to indicate the kinds of concerns that led up to the request for support and the kind of information the profession needs about the nurse practitioner movement.

The stated objectives of the conference were:

1. To provide information about newer models in psychiatric nursing practice for the profession as a whole and for its members, for interested agencies —public and private, national and local.
2. To provide information about legal aspects on problems of advanced and/or independent professional nursing practice.
3. To provide information about the economic aspects of practice and payment for services. To provide information about business management and public relations.
4. To provide information about acceptance and recognition of practitioners by patients and colleagues.
5. To provide information about ways of keeping current and intellectually stimulated in the various practice models (especially independent practice models).
6. To provide information about training programs or practices.
7. To work on issues to be resolved.
8. To identify innovations, trends, and projections for the future.
9. To identify sources of support.

At the time of the NIMH site visit on this grant proposal, the question of limiting the conference participants to mental health–psychiatric nurse practitioners was raised. Other nurse practitioner specialties are closely allied, and theories and modes of intervention among the various specialities have much in common. Also, psychiatric nursing as a specialty is confronted at the national policy level with demands for comprehensive health care. Thus, with the approval of the site visitor, it was decided to open up the conference invitation to generalists and representatives of other specialties as one way of looking at the nurse practitioner movement in the mainstream of health care.

PARTICIPANTS

Selection

In planning to meet the project objectives it was evident that representation from a wide variety of organizational and service practice arrangements would be useful. A wide geographic representation including both urban and rural practices was also required. In addition, different levels of academic preparation for practice needed to be represented. Representation from organized nursing was given priority in terms of the perspective this would provide. A limited number of representatives from programs training nurse practitioners were included to provide information about trends, educational preparation, and current research in this area of nursing practice.

Developing the selection criteria was not easy; there were differences of opinion on the Advisory Committee about the level of academic preparation required before one may call oneself or be called a nursing practitioner. Also, there was disagreement about including nurse practitioners other than mental health–psychiatric nurse practitioners. Membership in an ANA council of nurse practitioners was also urged as a criterion for participation.

Conferees

Selection of this diverse group of people for the conference was carefully planned, but in the end participation was mostly by coincidence and by accident. The literature was full of names of nurse practitioners who had written about their practices. It appeared that getting geographic practice representation and academic preparation representation would be easy, but most of the people who had written the early articles could not be located because they were not in practice in the places cited. Some were in universities and no longer carried a practice. Requests for information to executive secretaries of state boards of nursing and queries to friends in nursing were the most productive means of search, but changes in schedules and other commitments required filling the last vacancy a week before the conference. It would have been easy to find 40 people in full-time academic positions who carry patient loads either as part of their academic responsibilities or in addition to them, but full-time practicing nurses were hard to locate.

Half of the nurse practitioners selected were in psychiatric nursing and half represented other nursing specialities. Half were in private practice, and most were in some form of independent practice in that they carried their own case loads of clients for whom they were both responsible and accountable. Two faculty members represented nurse practitioner training programs. There were seven guests who participated actively as representatives of the American Nurses Association, the Division of Nursing of DHEW, and the Nurse Training Branch of NIMH, as well as members of the Advisory Committee of the conference and three invited resource people.

The participants were a group of articulate, assertive, highly committed nurse practitioners. They did not feel compelled to agree, and they were comfortable with differences and conflicts with the resource people and with each other. If one person's opinions differed from those of another and the discussion became heated, no anxious soul jumped in to make peace. In an unusual way they left each other free. Following are brief descriptions of the conference participants:

Sarah Ellen Archer

Sarah Ellen Archer is a community nurse practitioner with the nonprofit Nursing Dynamics Corporation. Other disciplines represented in the corporation are dietetics, physical therapy, pharmacy, and community mental health nursing. Dr. Archer practices in a senior center and in community pharmacies. She also teaches at the University of California, San Francisco. She sees about 35 clients a week for essentially long-term health care problems, although she sees clients with acute illnesses or minor injuries in the pharmacy setting. She joined this nursing movement because she wanted direct client contact, because she believes that nursing has important services for which we can ultimately be paid, because she wanted to be her own boss, because she was dissatisfied with dependent nurse roles, and because she disliked the disease focus of our health care system. A report of Dr. Archer's research in a typology of practice for community health nursing appears in the June 1975 issue of *Nursing Outlook.*

Maxine Bardach

Maxine Bardach of Northfield, Illinois, is in individual practice for profit. She does psychotherapy with individual adults and couples and is interested in doing more family therapy in the future. Her commitment to her very young family, her desire for more direct clinical experience, and her commitment to the concept of the nurse as a provider of primary care were basic to her going into private practice. She has built-in economic advice in that her husband is an economist.

Patty Brandner

Patty Brandner is a mental health therapist in a partnership that was organized for profit, Counseling Associates in Dallas, Texas. This is a loose partnership of four people who each have offices in their own homes but who contract for services with Women for Change and who work with the Women's Health Coalition; they work closely with two other nurses and a social worker in independent practice. Her clients are mostly women with whom she does individual and family counseling, especially in the areas of child rearing, sexuality, and crisis, including rape. She also consults with colleagues in other disciplines and other agencies. Ms. Brandner began practicing independently in 1959 when she initiated childbirth education classes and began taking people in crisis into her home. Her purpose in going to graduate school was to broaden the base of support of her independence. See the September 1974 *American Journal of Nursing* for a description of her women's group series.

Kathleen Brown

Kathleen Brown is a family nurse practitioner and an instructor in the Family Nurse Practitioner and Pediatric Nurse Practitioner Programs at Tulane University in New Orleans. She works jointly with physicians and performs health screening, health education, and management of chronically ill patients or patients with acute minor illnesses. She sought an independent practice role because of her dissatisfaction with jobs in which she functioned at a low level of authority and responsibility.

Evelyn M. Chapman

Evelyn M. Chapman practices in northwestern Wyoming. She is a family nurse practitioner in a profit-making venture providing health care in rural areas that are economically unable to support a physician. She treats all types of health care problems within the range of her skills in a large practice comprised of ranchers, oilfield workers, and construction workers.

Jay Croley

At the time of her selection, Jay Croley was in half-time private practice and was employed by the Santa Clara County Mental Health Center in California. Her private practice was an individual profit-making venture. She also worked on a fee-for-service basis for psychiatrists and taught on a fee basis at a number of colleges. She essentially uses Gestalt therapy methods with nonpsychotic adults (except for family therapy) who are interested in changing their life styles. Her clients are mostly middle-class urban women. She does not work with people who want hospitalization or medication. She went into private practice because "it is the only way to be paid appropriately for my skill and . . . the only way to have total control over my practice and to make direct contacts between me and my patients." Jay has a master's degree in medical-surgical nursing and has done further work in psychiatric nursing at the University of California, San Francisco; she has a second master's degree in counseling psychology from the University of California at Berkeley. She had a part-time practice for more than 5 years in Bangladesh and for 3 years in Cairo, besides holding both education and service positions in this country.

Lorene Fischer

Dr. Lorene Fischer is director of the psychiatric–mental health nursing program at Wayne State University in Detroit. During the last 5 years she has been involved in working with graduates of the Wayne program who are trying to establish roles as primary caretakers within various kinds of health care agencies. She has been looking particularly at the kinds of constraints these nurses are subject to and at the implications these constraints might have for the program. Most recently she has been involved in interdisciplinary planning and development of nursing clinics. She is working on this within the framework of the Wayne State University mandatory service clinic which will open in 1978. A side issue of this project is studying and planning for the kinds of nursing clinics that will meet the needs of inner-city residents in terms of health needs not now being met and the kinds of clients to be served.

Sharon Gedan

Sharon Gedan, currently of Los Angeles, was in individual practice ("hopefully for profit") in Honolulu. In addition to individual and group psychotherapy, she did sex, rape, preabortion, and couples' counseling. At another level of practice she provided consultation to health agencies and taught crisis techniques to nurses and auxiliary workers. She went into independent practice because she was not adequately compensated while working as a therapist and because she wanted to demonstrate that a nurse could compete in a downtown urban area.

Maddy Gerrish

Maddy Gerrish of Bedford, Massachusetts, is associated with profit and nonprofit organizations: Expansion, Inc., and Expansion Foundation, Inc. Expansion is a comprehensive mental health center in which Ms. Gerrish and a partner employ 16 consultants on either a full-time or part-time basis. She went into independent practice because of disillusionment with institutional practice of mental health. Her group sees about 300 middle-class suburban clients a week and deals with the entire range of psychiatric problems.

Mary Gray

Mary Gray is a family nurse practitioner on a part-time basis for the community known as Little Italy, Arkansas. She is a full-time faculty member at the School of Nursing, Univeristy of Arkansas. The families for whom she provides primary nursing service live in a rural area 40 miles from other health services. Her clients are a closely knit ethnic group ranging in age from 2 to 75 years. Her clients are required to find a physician who agrees to work with her before being accepted into her case load. This policy promotes care in referral, but more important it structures relationships for comprehensive health care right from the beginning. She is acting on her belief that all nurses should practice and that practitioners should be the leaders in nursing as they are in other professions.

Jocelyn A. Greenidge

Jocelyn A. Greenidge and two partners, Mary F. Kohnke and Ann R. Zimmern, are in a nonprofit partnership they have named Community Nurse Practitioners. They offer a full range of nursing services from infancy to old age. They work mostly with middle-aged and middle-income clients, with a slight predominance of women. They offer 24-hour-a-day service in the Stuyvesant Town area of New York City. These partners have written a book, *Independent Nurse Practitioner,* published by Trainex Press, that they use in lieu of a policy manual in guiding practice. They went into private practice because of their powerlessness to practice professional nursing under present institutional policies and under the new New York State Practice Act.

Leanne Halfman

Leanne Halfman is now on the faculty of Purdue University, but when she was identified for possible membership in this group she was a school nurse practitioner in Gary, Indiana. She is teaching physical assessment of adults and children to diploma and associate-degree registered nurses in a 2-year program leading to a baccalaureate degree who will then be considered nurse practitioners. Ms. Halfman and a colleague are in the process of setting up a part-time practice as nurse practitioners with hospital employees and university students.

Sister Carolita Hart

Sister Carolita Hart is a family nurse practitioner at the North West Family Health Center in Salt Lake City, Utah. She practices in economically depressed areas, seeking people who have difficulty getting into the traditional health care system. Her clients include Chicanos, Blacks, American Indians, and Caucasians. Sister Carolita carries a general case load, with a heavy mental health emphasis. She practices independently with physician backup.

Mary Alice Hauser

Mary Alice Hauser is in the independent practice of nursing at the Iowa Veterans Home in Marshalltown, Iowa. She provides individual therapy, group therapy, family therapy, crisis intervention, and consultation with clients and their families. She also participates in the in-service program at the home. Her clients are over 65 years old and are mostly men from rural communities in Iowa. There are 500 residents in this community of veterans, and she works on the basis of referrals from among this population. Veterans and their families are referred to her essentially for psychosocial therapeutic intervention. She and other nurses at the Iowa Veterans Home worked out this referral method as part of a broad reorganization of the nursing program to improve the delivery of health care and to eliminate some of the constraints placed on professional nursing practice by a bureaucratic system.

Marian Havlovic

Marian Havlovic is in the private practice of psychiatric nursing for profit. She works in Chicago and does individual and family counseling utilizing primarily the modalities of crisis intervention, short-term psychotherapy, and group psychotherapy. Sixty percent of her clients have metastatic carcinoma and are receiving ambulatory chemotherapy. The remaining 40 percent have benign hematologic disorders. She sees 10 to 20 clients per week.

Gertrude Isaacs

Dr. Gertrude Isaacs works for the well-known Frontier Nursing Service in the Appalachian region of Kentucky. She is well known in psychiatric circles as one of the first nurses to have a doctoral degree in nursing as well as for her association with the NIMH Training Branch in Nursing during the critical time of growth in psychiatric nursing. The Frontier Nursing Service provides health care management of a primarily rural population of 15,000 to 20,000 with families in low socioeconomic groups. Care is provided in homes, district clinics, and a hospital.

Nancy Keller

Nancy Keller practices in a partnership for profit named Nursing Care and Consultation, Ltd., from Tucson, Arizona. We say "from" Tucson because the two nurses in this partnership are often flying or driving over Arizona and the western states providing, in addition to nursing care, practice in techniques, health education, a large volume of consultation in research staff development, health care program development, and proposal formulation. In the 2 years of their practice the partners have had 125 to 150 clients of both sexes from the middle class in the middle-aged and retired groups. Ms. Keller was prompted to go into independent practice because she was confident that the theoretical frameworks she used in the academic setting would be useful in practice but had no time or opportunity to find out precisely how or why. Articles by Dr. Keller have appeared in recent issues of *The Journal of Nursing Service Administration.*

Karlene Kerfoot

Karlene Kerfoot of Iowa City is in part-time individual private practice for profit. Most of her clients are women who have sexual dysfunction problems, although she occasionally has a male patient and sometimes treats couples with a cotherapist. She carries ten open cases and has three to five on the waiting list. She works full time as a nurse practitioner with her own case load and as a colleague with all other therapists at the Cedar Rapids Mental Health Center.

Lucille Kinlein

Lucille Kinlein is in independent practice in Washington, D.C. She celebrated 25 years in nursing by hanging out her shingle in testimony of nursing's reaching the fullness of professional maturity. She is nationally recognized as a master teacher and has an appointment at the faculty of Georgetown University School of Nursing. Her paper "Independent Nurse Practitioner" appeared in the January 1972 issue of *Nursing Outlook.*

Mary Ann Lewis

Mary Ann Lewis directs the Family Nurse Practitioner Program at the University of California, Los Angeles. She also practices in a women's cancer screening clinic, in an internal medicine clinic, and in a diabetic service doing total examination including laboratory data and problem list. She sees patients in all economic brackets, both men and women, from the greater Los Angeles area. She works closely with social workers, nutritionists, and physicians.

Ingeborg Mauksch

Dr. Ingeborg Mauksch is a family nurse practitioner of the School of Medicine faculty and in the Family Care Center at the University of Missouri, which is nonprofit. Her patient load includes the entire range of illness and health problems in all age groups of both sexes. She is also chairperson of the American Nurses' Association Commission on Nursing Practice and is a frequent contributor to the nursing literature.

Nancy Milio

Dr. Nancy Milio works in a Boston-based nonprofit corporation, Alternatives in Health Care. She works with others in many other disciplines both health- and nonhealth-related, and the corporation has group clients in other regions of the United States. She and her colleagues provide consultation in the organization of health services, education and training, content development, program development, and evaluation in health service delivery. Dr. Milio was one of the first nurses to write of her practice. She is author of the book *9226 Kercheval: The Storefront That Did Not Burn.*

Elaine I. Nielsen

Elaine I. Nielsen of Beresford, South Dakota, is in a "hopefully profitable" individual practice in a community of 7500 people where there is no physician. She works with preoperative and postoperative patients in their homes, she deals with physical and emotional emergencies that occur in the community, she teaches self-help classes, and she teaches babysitters how to babysit, among many other functions. She sees 50 to 75 patients per week in all age groups. Her clients represent essentially middle-class females and males. Although her clients live within a 10-mile radius, she travels 26,000 miles per year. She went into private practice 18 years ago because of the desperate need in her community for health care. She has a real grasp of the problems of going into independent practice; she has many suggestions for those who are interested and has had many of the same experiences that beginning practitioners are having today.

Janelle Smith Ramsburg

Janelle Smith Ramsburg is in private practice for profit in Kansas City, Missouri. She does individual, group, and family therapy. In addition, she teaches courses in group therapy and transactional analysis for the University of Missouri and does some consultation with social and health agencies. Her clients are middle- and upper-middle-class men and women ranging from their teens to old age. She has medical backup from a psychiatrist for medication and for hospitalization if necessary. She decides whether to follow patients in the hospital or ask the psychiatrist to do so. After discharge, patients return to her practice. When patients are referred to her by family physicians, she arranges for medications as needed through them. She went into private practice because she wanted the opportunity to do what she knew how to do, because other therapists encouraged her to do so, and because she was tired of hospital and agency "games."

Janice Ruffin

Janice Ruffin has an individual practice within the Connecticut Mental Health Center in New Haven. She provides individual and group therapy for patients referred to the Psychotherapy Unit of the Center. Her clients are young adults, adults, and the middle-aged, with a full range of psychiatric diagnoses, although most have characterologic problems manifested in neurotic behavior. Over the years she found she did not require the structure characteristic of many psychiatric settings, and she finds a great deal of gratification in functioning autonomously with appropriate resources (eg, medical backup) available to her.

Ada Shannon

Ada Shannon is a pediatric nurse practitioner working with the Kaiser-Permanente Medical Group and Hospital Foundation for a profit partnership of physicians. She works in the Santa Clara unit. She performs complete physical assessments, well-baby checks, and evaluation and screening relative to development and nutrition, as well as a wide range of disease-prevention and health-promotion functions. Her clients of both sexes range in age from 2 months to 3 years. She sees 12 to 16 children and infants per day. She went into this work because she couldn't resist the challenge and because her pioneer instincts told her that professional nursing was headed in this direction.

Nancy C. Talley

Nancy C. Talley of Tampa, Florida, is in both individual practice for profit and practice with a nonprofit community mental health center attached to a hospital. She does marriage and family counseling, individual and group psychotherapy, and evaluation and therapy with children, as well as community consultation and workshops. Her current case load is 36 patients ranging in age from 18 months to 64 years.

Lynn Theuer

Lynn Theuer went into business November 3, 1975, in a profit-making corporate structure named Nursing Consultation, Inc. She has two nurse partners. They do individual and group educational services. She was prompted to go into independent practice because of the need for psychotherapy in clients' homes and because a partnership was available to offer 24-hour services in a feasible manner.

Sally Tripp

Sally Tripp of Amherst, Massachusetts, is director of the Nurse Practitioner Project at the University of Massachusetts. She was one of the early participants in the nurse practitioner movement.

Her work with the interdisciplinary group in the medical clinic at the Massachusetts General Hospital to establish the nurse practitioner program there has been well publicized in medical and nursing journals.

Josephine Vander Meer

Josephine Vander Meer is an independent nurse practitioner working in a family practice clinic. Her practice is limited to sex offenders, victims of sexual abuse, and families of both offenders and victims. She performs crisis intervention, intake interviews, family assessment, and individual and family counseling. Much of her practice is carried out on the telephone, since many of these clients resist clinic appointments. She also does a great deal of work in clients' homes. She and three other members make up a team for this program, and they all take calls so one person is available to go to a client in crisis 24 hours a day, 7 days a week. Dr. Vander Meer has just finished her doctoral work, in which she made an in-depth study of the adolescent rape victim.

Margaret Wacker

Margaret Wacker of New York City is a family therapist in individual practice for profit. Most of her clients are lower middle-class couples, although some women are seen individually. She went into independent private practice because she wanted to function at a graduate professional level without the limitations of hospital or clinic nursing departments. She has a psychiatrist for medical back-up, such as drug evaluations, and she is able to receive third-party payments on the psychiatrist's signature. Like other members in this category, she cited as her first problem the educating of other nurses, as well as those in other disciplines, to the fact that she can give quality therapy and can function independently.

Carolyn Whitaker

Carolyn Whitaker is in family practice as an employee of a physician. She sees an average of 40 clients per day who have problems related to preventive health, primary illness, or chronic disease. Her dissatisfaction with a health care delivery system that prevented the practice of nursing and thwarted its potential for providing health care was basic to her entering graduate study to become prepared as a family nurse practitioner. She works in a rural area because opportunities for her are greater in this kind of setting.

Carolyn Williams

Carolyn Williams is a research nurse who has been involved in evaluation studies of the Faculty Nurse Practitioner Program in the state of North Carolina. These studies have included the implications of conducting a training program with the aim of preparing individuals to respond to problems of health care delivery within a defined area, as well as the potential influence of practice setting characteristics on development of expanded roles. Dr. Williams is on the faculty of the University of North Carolina.

Virginia Williams

Virginia Williams is in the individual practice for profit of family nursing, with an office in McHenry, Illinois. She serves several small towns. Most of her clients have long-term problems that require family support and adaptation. She does have some paraplegics and 15 or 20 children in her case load. Her clientele is essentially rural and middle class. She confers with clients' physicians when indicated, but otherwise she does not work with any individual physician. Several insurance companies, including CNA, Teachers Retirement, New York Life, American Mutual, Home Insurance, Mutual of New York, State Bank Trust Fund, Metropolitan Life, as well as Medicaid (through the public aid department) provide third-party payment for her services.

PROGRAM

The conference program was planned with input from the participants. This was accomplished by sending to the participants a list of possible topics to be discussed in the small work groups and asking them to rank the topics in order of importance or interest to them. While there was a great deal of disagreement with regard to the importance of specific subjects, there was sufficient consensus to plan for 12 work group sessions, with the four sessions that received highest priority being repeated. In addition, two sessions were planned so that practitioners might get together to discuss how they could develop mechanisms for communicating with one another in matters of common interest. A copy of the program is included in the Appendixes.

In addition to the program input solicited from the participants, the participants were asked to complete a lengthy questionnaire to provide information regarding themselves and their practices. From these questionnaires, a brief profile was developed for each participant, statistical summaries of the characteristics of the group were made, and critical incidents illustrating the participants' practices with their clients and their relationships with other professionals were abstracted. This information from the questionnaires was distributed to the participants prior to the conference so that they would have some knowledge of the composition of the group and the kinds of experiences others had had. Following input from the participants, the conference program (Appendix A) was developed around three major themes: the nurse practitioner movement within the whole of health services, the legal issues for the nurse practitioner, and the issues of economics. Minor themes worked into the program were identification of health needs, clientele to be served, defining the scope of services, strategies for selling services to others, and forms of association with other professionals. Concerns about policy and research in the nurse practitioner movement were also included. One minor theme called "Loose Thinkers and Dreamers" was added to provide discussion on where the future lies and what the growing edge of the movement might be. As noted earlier, and as is apparent in the report, there was great variation in depth and scope in dealing with the issues.

EVALUATION

The conference was held in the middle of an airlines strike. People came late and left early, and some never got there. Speakers who arrived late made constant program revision necessary.

For some participants it was their first meeting with nurse practitioners. Two sets of objectives emerged: an urgent personal set and an external set imposed by the conference staff. Some participants were more experienced in practice, sophisticated in business matters, and conversant with the politics of state and federal health care policy than were others. This resulted in objectives being dealt with on many levels. In addition, some objectives of the conference did not seem relevant to the concerns of some practitioners.

All participants dealt at some length with a four-page postconference evaluation form sent to them 2 months after the conference ended. Evaluations ranged all the way from ecstasy about the usefulness of the conference to anger because it was a complete waste of time. Some participants had found the resource people useful, and others felt that they had been talked down to. Almost all participants wanted to have other conferences at which personal problems could be presented, at which nursing data could be shared and examined, and at which issues could be discussed in depth. There were many suggestions for conducting future conferences.

One significant observation coming out of the evaluations is that some participants had already developed formal conceptualizations about nurse practitioner practice and would not consider the ideas of others. Some were more open and exploring in their approach. Others were trying to assess directions, meanings, and perspectives for nursing in the health care system, and a few were looking for guidance.

The nurse practitioners also perceived that there were wide differences in sophistication and experience among the participants, and they wished to meet with members who were at their own level. While it did not emerge as a theme in the evaluations, the tremendous differences in outlook and approach between mental health–psychiatric nurse participants and participants in other nursing disciplines were mentioned; these were also noted by conference staff and resource people.

One of the greatest values of the conference was the informal contacts and opportunities to talk with experienced leaders in the field.

One of the greatest drawbacks noted by participants was lack of structure and organization for getting the work of the conference done. What the conference staff saw as freedom to explore the issues was perceived by some to be poor organization, poor group leadership, and lack of good direction. There was also great variability of response regarding the usefulness of the resource people.

The following chapters attempt to summarize the work, the concerns, and the evaluations of this 2-day conference of nurse practitioners.

CHAPTER 2

One Perspective on the Nurse Practitioner Movement

Catherine M. Norris

A great complex of values, situations, and events contributed to the evolution of professional nursing and the emergence of the nurse practitioner. But what ideas or events in nursing itself supported or promoted nursing practices that made the role of the nurse practitioner a viable alternative for professional nurses today? Nursing history has essentially been biographical history, and a history of ideas might make the evolution of nursing more understandable. We need to examine the following questions: Where and when were its guiding ideas introduced into nursing? What ideas were picked up and developed, and which ones were lost? Which surfaced again at a much later date? How were the ideas developed? How long did it take? How did they affect nursing practice and health care? Who initiated ideas and who developed them? How did the ideas become powerful or influential enough to cause change?

First, what events or situations brought about the widespread acceptance of the expanded role of the professional nurse? There is no shortage of possibilities. A statement was issued by the Academy of Nursing to the effect that "the Nurse Practitioner approach is regarded as the most effective, least costly way to solve one of the major health problems, the uneven distribution of health care personnel and facilities. The nurse-practitioner, it was judged, is the logical person to provide the primary care so critically needed in rural areas and in the ghettos."[1] One can read into this statement a rational problem-solving, decision-making approach to unmet health needs. But we remember that in 1970 the American Medical Association (AMA) planned unilateral action to train 70,000 nurses to work under physicians in assistant roles. In addition, the AMA was at that time supporting the proliferation of programs for preparing assistant physicians, a program that would put distance between nurses and patients as well as between nurses and physicians and would move the nurse down one step in the power and prestige structure of health agencies. Rather than being a rational planned change, is there an element of backlash in the nurse practitioner movement?

Coming at this particular time, does the nurse practitioner movement perhaps reflect the contribution of the women's movement in making nurses conscious of their human and creative potential, in improving woman's self-concept, in offering possibilities for significance, status, and economic equality, and in making us aware of the self-defeating aspects of alienated behaviors?[2,3]

Is the nurse practitioner movement an aspect of the drive of all health care groups to fulfill their manifest destiny? Both nonprofessional and professional health care personnel are concerned with delineating their spheres of control in the health care system. Some of these groups have claimed some of nursing's prerogatives. In order to survive, must nursing invade the territory of others or carve out new functions? Or is the movement related to the social theme of activism as one way to achieve power and thereby reduce feelings of helplessness and powerlessness?

Is the movement perhaps a response to being trapped between physicians and the upward-moving licensed practical nurse group? Is it a response to the administrative definition of nursing by agencies, with the recently added threat of institutional licensure? Is it partly in response to the actions of health agencies in usurping the powers of state boards of nursing, restricting the freedom to practice professional nursing and acting as the responsible agents for nursing practice?

Abdellah[4] and Keller [5] draw a vivid picture of the events in nursing following World War II that placed licensed practical nurses, aides, and other ancillary workers between nurse and patient while creating a variety of coordinating and supervising functions for nurses that moved them even farther away from the patients. They suggest that the nurse practitioner movement is a way back to the patient. Keller[5] adds a note of urgency in identifying the movement as an effort to regain and maintain the profession's birthright.

Is the movement related to anticipation or recognition of the fact that professional nursing as we once knew it is at an end?[6] The day when the nurse was as important to the patient's recovery as the physician is already gone. The discovery of sulfanilamides and penicillin opened the way to cure through pharmacology, as well as surgery, and other technologic advances, which rapidly made nursing obsolescent and care by the physician all-important.

Is the nurse practitioner movement a response to federal legislation on professional standards that gives medicine the responsibility for health care, leaving professional nursing and direct payment for nursing services out of health care plans (Medicare and Health Maintenance Organizations) and national health insurance plans, supporting nursing education and research only as a poor fifth cousin of medicine?

Is the nurse practitioner movement a reaction to the last in a long series of moves by medicine to turn over some of its functions to nursing while still maintaining all authority for the function? In other words, is it a reaction against further subjugation or a less helpless, more prestigious form of subjugation?

Is the nurse practitioner movement a backlash to further economic exploitation by physicians and hospital administrators? Is it a rejection of directors of nursing who, in order to survive, must implement the controls, policies, and values of business administration rather than free nurses and support them to function professionally? Put another way, is it a reaction to hospital politics, where nurses are betrayed by those in the profession who hold or supposedly hold the power?

Is the movement the culmination of the concerted drive that began in 1948 with the recommendation of the Brown report related to collegiate education for professional nursing? Is it a consequence of our readiness for theory-based professional practice? Is it related to the recognition that after years of work on the concept of clinical specialization we find that specialization is synonomous with practice, ie, one simply cannot remain a specialist and function only as a teacher or coordinator or administrator. Or did the nurse practitioner movement come about through gradual evolution as the direction in which we were heading all the time? On at least one level (that involving ideas and their application to practice) the movement required 30 years of intensive work by scholars and practitioners of nursing. If this work had not been done, the nurse practitioner movement could not have become a stable alternative for resolving society's health care problems or the problems of professional nursing.

FERMENT IN PSYCHIATRIC NURSING

It was 30 years ago that the seeds for radical change in nursing practice were sown, and the early efforts came in psychiatric nursing. In 1944 only 54 percent of the nation's nursing schools offered courses in psychiatric nursing.[7] Psychiatric nursing was rarely required for licensure and 13 states offered no course of any kind in psychiatric nursing.[8] Only 5 of every 100 generic nursing students were enrolled in collegiate programs. Early in World War II the American Psychiatric Association became concerned about the decrease in the number of nurses working in psychiatry and the increase in the number of mental hospitals.[8] Nurses in the armed services during the war were confronted with psychiatric casualty problems, and they had no experience in nursing patients with emotional difficulties.

In 1945 the nurses returning from the armed services (where they had had great responsibility and authority in patient care) were dissatisfied with civilian nursing practice and with their own nursing skills.[9] They had the money, under the GI bill, to get an education, and they demanded education in nursing. Up to that time there had been no clinical postgraduate courses except those offered in specialty hospitals as supervised work experience. The nine collegiate programs for graduate nurses prepared them for functional roles only, but the need for clinical expertise had become an issue.[10]

In 1946 funds were made available to colleges under the Mental Health Act for education in psychiatric nursing,[11] and functional role programs were adjusted to include psychiatric nursing courses, although there was often little change in emphasis on the functional role because of the existing assumption that education for nursing practice was terminal at the diploma level. But the increases in the amount of support and the number of programs supported gave psychiatric nurse faculty members an edge in developing the discipline. A 1945 editorial in the *American Journal of Nursing* may have a familiar ring: "Advanced clinical courses are still in their experimental stage, but their proponents have the zeal of pioneers."[9] Faculty in other nursing specialty areas, saddled with teaching, administration, and supervision programs, did not have the same opportunity until passage of the Nurse Training Act in 1964.

GRADUATE EDUCATION IN CLINICAL NURSING

Until almost the middle 1950s advanced clinical nursing education was essentially at the baccalaureate level for qualified nurses, and a qualified nurse was one who had graduated from a state-approved diploma school. The *American Journal of Nursing Index* does not list Graduate Education as a subject heading until 1952, and the National League for Nursing (NLN) started to publish a list of accredited graduate programs in nursing only in 1960. How short is our professional history.

NURSING AS A PROFESSION: PRINCIPLES UNDERLIE PRACTICE

What were the ideas that permitted at least some nurses to become professional practitioners of nursing? One idea was that nursing was an applied science rather than a set of tasks, activities, and routines carried out within a set of rules. This idea was developed around the application of scientific and nursing principles. While the idea was advanced by Robb in 1893,[12] by Van Blarcom in 1923,[13] and by others, it was Martha Ruth Smith[14] who through her work with students and the wide adoption of her nursing text made one of the greatest contributions in moving nursing away from the tasks and activities orientation. Her work provided the model for other texts, using scientific principles to organize the subject matter of nursing. One or two of these texts remain in print and in use today. For the first time nurses were provided with a systematic way of approaching and using a body of knowledge for understanding and meaning as well as for developing guides to action.

CLINICAL NURSING SPECIALIST

In 1944 the Committee to Study Postgraduate Clinical Nursing Courses of the National League for Nursing Education advanced the concept of a new type of nurse—the clinical nursing specialist.[15] Prior to that time preparation for nursing leadership was found in teaching and administration through philosophy and methods courses. The clinical nurse specialist was described as being an expert practitioner who had developed expertise through supervised clinical practice. Up to that time no academic program beyond the diploma level required supervised clinical practice in nursing. In 1953 the NLN again took the lead in supporting and publishing a study[16] that moved psychiatric nursing out of tasks, activities, and employment roles to conceptual terms. In 1956 a national conference to deal with education for this emerging role was held in Williamsburg, Virginia, under the auspices of the National League for Nursing.[17]

CONCEPTUAL SKILLS

The need for conceptual skills as a requirement for expert practice was made explicit by Hildegard Peplau in her book *Interpersonal Relations in Nursing* published in 1952.[18] The skills of analysis and synthesis required for concept building and the ability to operationalize concepts and to move from literal to symbolic levels of thinking were taught widely by Peplau, who is a master teacher, and by graduates of her program. Dorothy Gregg developed the concept of anxiety while she was a student in Peplau's program, as well as the concept of reassurance, both of which were published during the 1950s.[19,20] Tudor's study, "A Sociopsychiatric Nursing Approach to Intervention in a Problem of Mutual Withdrawal on a Mental Hospital Ward," which used the conceptual approach, was published in 1952.[21] Because of their quality these three articles are classics, and they remain useful today. Other leaders in promoting the conceptual approach to nursing were Shirley Burd and Margaret Marshall,[22] Loretta Zderad and Helen Belcher,[23] and Carolyn Carlson.[24] With their work the content and method of psychiatric nursing began to take shape. It was only after 1964, when federal support became available in other areas of nursing, that work was begun in developing clinical content in pediatric and medical-surgical nursing.

INDEPENDENT FUNCTIONS

In 1957 Frances Reiter Kreuter delineated the dependent and independent functions in nursing practice.[25] The introduction of the idea of independent functions was important to nursing at a time when physicians were making a fairly general practice of ordering nursing care as part of the medical orders. It helped nursing to focus on its unique contribution to health care and provided hope for a more productive, creative future in professional nursing practice. There followed increasing revision and expansion: Lydia Hall in 1957,[26] Loretta Ford in 1967,[27] Charles Lewis and Barbara Resnick in 1967,[28,29] and Lucille Kinlein in 1972[30] contributed four different kinds of practice models wherein nursing practice was independent. Different kinds of collaborative arrangements with medicine for the medical aspects of care were developed.

NURSING PROCESSES: CONTENT AND METHODOLOGY OF NURSING

In 1952 Peplau identified the nursing processes of assessment, diagnosis, and intervention as the methodology of nursing.[18] In 1955 Lyle Saunders, a sociologist student of nursing, identified assessment as a major characteristic of nursing practice,[31] and Rozella Schlotfeldt used the term in her 1962 definition of nursing.[32] Mary Lou Lyon was using a nursing history at Emory University in 1960. Lesnick and Anderson identified nursing diagnosis as a nursing responsibility in the 1947 edition of their book *Legal Aspects of Nursing*.[33] In 1953 Vera Fry,[34] followed by Gertrude Hornung,[35] Wilda Chambers,[36] and others,[37,38] contributed to the development of the nursing diagnostic process. In 1964 Norris synthesized a model for the nursing process based on the assumption that the nursing process is the unique content of nursing.[39] Mary Thomas and Rosemary Prince developed a scholarly elucidation of nursing diagnosis that was published in 1965.[40] Faye McCain[41] and Mae McPhetridge[42] did some of the early work on assessment. Hildegard Peplau,[43,44] Marion Kalkman,[45] Gwen Tudor,[21] Dorothy Gregg,[19,20] and Theresa Muller[46] did much of the early work on psychiatric nursing intervention. Yura and Walsh have also made significant contributions to the elucidation of the nursing process.[47] While the development of the theory of the nursing process is still in its infancy, it provides nurses with a common body of knowledge, a known methodology about which to communicate, and outcomes that can be evaluated and from which it is possible to generate testable hypotheses.

NURSING IS THERAPEUTIC . . . NURSING IS THERAPY

In 1952 Peplau wrote that nursing is therapeutic and that some skilled nursing is therapy.[18] In 1953 June Mellow talked about nurses' involvement in therapy, and by 1956 she was using the terms nursing therapy and nurse therapist.[48] This presaged an overlapping of the roles and functions of nursing with the roles of other professional disciplines where there was already considerable overlap. It raised expectations and set the stage for testing and developing collaborative relationships with other disciplines that would to a great extent replace dependent and articulating relationships. This has progressed to the point where several participants in this conference expressed indignation that they have not been given hospital privileges. This is far removed from the time when nurses hedged about calling nursing therapeutic and called the nursing process problem-solving skills long after it was clear that we were on the way to developing our own discipline.

NURSING THEORY

The decade 1965–1975 has been called the decade of content and theory development. In 1959 Dorothy Johnson introduced the use of the idea of homeostasis as a useful theory for guiding nursing practice.[49] Ida Orlando's book *The Dynamic Nurse Patient Relationship,* on which the Yale University faculty built nursing practice theory, was published in 1958.[50] The first of Martha Rogers' three books, *Educational Revolution in Nursing,* came out in 1961.[51] Florence Wald,[52] Donna Diers,[53] Hildegard Peplau,[54] Betty Highley,[55] Rosemary Ellis,[56] Jeanne Quint Benoliel,[57] Imogene King,[58] and Ada Jacox[59] have all contributed significantly to theories for nursing. Margaret Kaufmann[60] and Lillian Pierce,[61] to name only two of a large group, have studied the usefulness of systems theory for nursing. Theory development is a natural sequel to concept work and a natural precursor to research in nursing. All three are necessary if the study of nursing is to be systematic and internally consistent and is to yield testable hypotheses and if a body of scientific nursing knowledge is to be realized.

The recognition that the organization of medical knowledge dichotomized patients and prevented a health care focus was important. Nursing had to search for ways to unify care so that people could be seen in their wholeness and humanness. Leadership for integration of public health, nutrition, orthopedic, and mental health concepts was exercised by the National League for Nursing Education in the 1930s and was continued by the National League for Nursing in the 1950s. Ruth Gilbert and Edna Fritz were leaders and innovators in this endeavor in the late 1940s and early 1950s. Faye Abdellah's doctoral work, in which she developed the 21-problems approach to nursing, gave impetus to the search for organizing themes for nursing practice.[62] Following in fairly rapid succession, other theoretical frames of reference were selected from other disciplines for use in nursing. These included family dynamics, Murphy's and Maslow's hierarchy of human needs, Erikson's concepts of growth and development and the health–illness continuum, Dunn's concept of high-level wellness, and adaptation theory. Most recently, the nursing process has been used with one or more other theories to give direction to nursing in terms of health promotion, recognizing and utilizing patients' strengths, and delineating differences between illness and health.

With an organized body of knowledge at hand, as well as expertise in the methods of making knowledge operational on behalf of patients and clients, the ideas necessary for the development of the nurse practitioner movement began to emerge. The concept of commitment was reworked, with Sister Madeleine Clemence providing leadership for this task. The ideas of responsibility, rights,[63] and accountability[64] were revised. Standards were reviewed, and the concept of certification for practice was introduced and developed. When we were ready, we demanded direct access to clients and patients.[65]

With awareness of the difficulties of finding one's way through the dehumanized health care system and with an increasingly receptive attitude to consumer influence on health care,[66] nursing brought the concept of the ombudsman into play; however, because of the legal connotations and the limitations of this role, the concept of advocacy[67,68] emerged as the role for nursing. Kosik spelled out this function in 1972, adding a new dimension to nursing for a huge ambulatory as well as institutionalized client population. Patient advocacy, consumer-controlled care, and health and growth promotion are gaining strength as important nursing concepts of health care.

These are only a few of the ideas and a few of the people who made it possible for us to be here today and to pick up the important work of making our real contribution to health care.

REFERENCES

1. Kellog N: Special report: how nursing leaders see your expanding role. RN 38:31, April 1975
2. Lamb KT: Freedom for our sisters; freedom for ourselves: nursing confronts social changes. Nurs Forum 12(4):328, 1973
3. Ashley JA: Nursing and early feminism. Am J Nurs 75:1465, September 1975
4. Abdellah FG: Evaluation of nursing as a profession: perspective in manpower development. Int Nurs Rev 19:219, 1972
5. Keller NS: The why's and what's of private practice. J Nurs Admin 5:12, June 1975
6. Wollowick AL: Will the nursing profession become extinct? Nurs Forum 9:408, 1970
7. National League for Nursing, Department of Studies: Nursing specialties in the curriculum. Am J Nurs 44:680, July 1944
8. Fitzsimmons LW: Facts and trends in psychiatric nursing. Am J Nurs 44:752, August 1944
9. Editor: Am J Nurs 45:878, November 1945
10. Favreau CH: Existing needs in psychiatric nursing. Am J Nurs 45:716, September 1945
11. News item: Am J Nurs 46:637, September 1946
12. Robb IH: Nursing: Its Principles and Practice for Hospital and Private Use. New York, Macmillan, 1893
13. Van Blarcom CC: Obstetrical Nursing. New York, Macmillan, 1923
14. Smith MR: Principles of Nursing Care. Philadelphia, Lippincott, 1936
15. National League for Nursing, Committee to Study Post-graduate Clinical Nursing Courses: Advanced course in psychiatric nursing. Am J Nurs 44:683, July 1944
16. Fagin CM: Nurses' rights. Am J Nurs 75:82, January 1975
17. National League for Nursing: Concepts in the Behavioral Sciences in Basic Nursing Education: Proceedings of the 1958 Regional Conferences on Psychiatric Nursing Education. New York, National League for Nursing, 1958
18. Peplau HE: Interpersonal Relations in Nursing. New York, Putnam, 1952
19. Gregg DE: Anxiety—a factor in nursing care. Am J Nurs 52:1363, November 1952
20. Gregg DE: Reassurance. Am J Nurs 55:171, February 1955
21. Tudor GE: A sociopsychiatric nursing approach to intervention in a problem of mutual withdrawal on a mental hospital ward. Psychiatry 15:193, May 1952
22. Burd SF, Marshall MA (eds): Some Clinical Approaches to Psychiatric Nursing. New York, Macmillan, 1963
23. Zderad LT, Belcher HC: Developing Behavioral Concepts in Nursing. Atlanta, Southern Regional Education board, 1968
24. Carlson CE (ed): Behavioral Concepts and Nursing Intervention. Philadelphia, Lippincott, 1970
25. Kreuter FR: What is good nursing care? Nurs Outlook 5:302, May 1957

26. Hall LE: The Loeb Center for Nursing and Rehabilitation, Montefiore Hospital and Medical Center, Bronx, New York. Int J Nurs Stud 6:81, July 1969
27. Ford LC, Silver HK: Physician's assistants. Part 3: the pediatric nurse practitioner at Colorado. Am J Nurs 67:1443, July 1967
28. Resnick BA: The Nursing Clinic: An Experiment in Ambulatory Patient Care. ANA Reg Clin Conf. New York, ANA, 1967, p 95
29. Lewis CE, Resnick BA: Nurse clinics and progressive ambulatory patient care. N Engl J Med 00:1239, 1967
30. Kinlein L: Independent nurse practitioner. Nurs Outlook 20:22, January 1972
31. Saunders L: The changing role of nurses, in Scott WR, Vokart EH (eds): Medical Care: Readings in the Sociology of Medical Institutions. New York, Wiley, 1966, p 437
32. Schlotfeldt R: Problems in the development of adequate criteria. Nurs Res 11:211, Fall 1962
33. Lesnick MJ, Anderson BE: Legal Aspects of Nursing. Philadelphia, Lippincott, 1947, p 352
34. Fry VS: The creative approach to nursing. Am J Nurs 53:301, March 1953
35. Hornung GJ: The nursing diagnosis—an exercise in judgment. Nurs Outlook 4:29, January 1956
36. Chambers W: Nursing diagnosis. Am J Nurs 62:102, November 1962
37. Bonny V, Rothberg J: Nursing Diagnosis and Therapy. New York, National League for Nursing, 1963
38. Komorita NI: Nursing diagnosis. Am J Nurs 63:83, December 1963
39. Norris CM: Toward a science of nursing—a method for developing unique content in nursing. Nurs Forum 3:10, 1964
40. Prince R, Durand M: Nursing diagnosis: process and decision. Nurs Forum 5:50, 1966
41. McCain RF: Nursing by assessment—not intuition. Am J Nurs 63:82, April 1965
42. McPhetridge LM: Nursing history: one means to personalize care. Am J Nurs 68:68, January 1968
43. Peplau HE: Historical development of psychiatric nursing (mimeographed). 1956
44. Peplau HE: Loneliness. Am J Nurs 55:1476, December 1955
45. Kalkman ME: What the psychiatric nurse should be educated to do. Psychiatr Q [Suppl], Part I, 1952
46. Muller TG: Nature and Direction of Psychiatric Nursing. Philadelphia, Lippincott, 1950
47. Yura H, Walsh MB: The Nursing Process, Assessing, Planning, Implementing, Evaluating. New York, Appleton, 1973
48. Colliton MA: The history of nursing theory: a reactionaire to the work of June Mellow. Perspect Psychiatr Care 3:10, 1965
49. Johnson DE: The nature of science of nursing. Nurs Outlook 7:291, May 1959
50. Orlando I: The Dynamic Nurse Patient Relationship. New York, Putnam, 1958
Rogers M: Educational Revolution in Nursing. New York, Macmillan, 1961

52. Wald FS, Leonard RC: Towards development of nursing practice theory. Nurs Res 13:309, Fall 1964
53. Diers D, Dye MC: Situation producing theory, in: Proceedings, Second Nursing Theory Conference, Kansas City, University of Kansas Medical Center, Department of Nursing Education, October 1969 p 73
54. Peplau H: Theory: the professional dimension. In Norris CM (ed): Proceedings, First Nursing Theory Conference, Kansas City, University of Kansas Medical Center, March 1969. Department of Nursing Education, 1969, p 33
55. Highley B: Defining Clinical Content—Graduate Nursing Programs: Maternal Child Health Nursing, Part I, Philosophy and Methodology. Boulder, Colorado, Western Interstate Commission for Higher Education, 1967
56. Ellis R: Characteristics of significant theories. Nurs Res 17:217, May–June 1968
57. Quint JC: Some thoughts on a theory of chronicity. In Norris CM (ed): Proceedings, First Nursing Theory Conference, Kansas City, University of Kansas Medical Center, March 1969, Department of Nursing Education, 1969, p 58
58. King I: Toward a Theory for Nursing. New York, Wiley, 1971
59. Jacox A: Theory construction in nursing: an overview. Nurs Res 23:4, January–February 1974
60. Kaufmann MA: A time, stress, perception model for theory development. In Norris CM (ed): Prodeedings, First Nursing Theory Conference, Kansas City, University of Kansas Medical Center, March 1969. Department of Nursing Education, p 23
61. Pierce L: General systems theory—an overview. In: Proceedings, Second Nursing Theory Conference, Kansas City, University of Kansas Medical Center, October 1969. Department of Nursing Education, 1969, p 73
62. Abdellah FG: Patient-centered Approaches to Nursing. New York, Macmillan, 1960
63. Fagin CM: Nurses' rights. Am J Nurs 75:82, January 1975
64. Maas M: Nurse autonomy and accountability. Nurs Forum 12:237, 1973
65. Norris CM: Direct access to the patient. Am J Nurs 70:1006, May 1970
66. Kramer M: The consumer's influence on health care. Nurs Outlook 20:574, September 1972
67. Kosik SH: Patient advocacy of fighting the system. Am J Nurs 72:694, April 1972
68. Nations WC: Nurse-lawyer is patient advocate. Am J Nurs 73:1039, June 1973

BIBLIOGRAPHY

Bowman RA, Culpepper RC: Power: Rx for change. Am J Nurs 74:1054, June 1974

Brown EL: Nursing for the Future. New York, Russell Sage, 1948

Brown MM: The epidemiological approach to the study of clinical nursing diagnosis. Nurs Forum 13:346, 1975

Dugan AB: Nursing autonomy: key to quality nurturance. Hosp Prog 51:47, April 1970

Gebbie KM, Lavin MA (eds): Classification of Nursing Diagnoses: Proceedings of the First National Conference held in St. Louis, October 15, 1973. St Louis, Mosby, 1975

Gebbie KM, Lavin MA: Classifying nursing diagnosis. Am J Nurs 74:250, February 1974

Gilbert R: The Public Health Nurse and Her Patient. Cambridge, Harvard University Press, 1951

Graves HH: Can nursing shed bureaucracy? Am J Nurs 71:490, March 1971

Johnson DE: The significance of nursing care. Am J Nurs 61:63, November 1961

National League for Nursing: The Education of the Clinical Specialist in Psychiatric Nursing. New York, National League for Nursing, 1958

Ozimek D, Yura H: Who Is the Nurse Practitioner? New York, National League for Nursing, 1975

Patient assessment: taking a patient's history (programmed instruction). Am J Nurs 74:293, February 1974

Payne SM: The evaluation of therapeutic care and clinical specialization in psychiatric nursing. Perspect Psychiatr Care 4:12, 1966

Platform of the American Nurses Association. New York, American Nurses Association, 1968

Ramphal M: Clinical and administrative judgment. Am J Nurs 72:1606, September 1962

Riehl JP, Roy C: Conceptual Models for Nursing Practice. New York, Appleton, 1974

Vaillot, Sister MC: Commitment to Nursing. Philadelphia, Lippincott, 1962

CHAPTER 3

Going into Practice

REASONS FOR GOING INTO PRACTICE

Nurses give a wide range of reasons for going into independent and private practice. There are many who wanted to meet a community need or unmet patient needs. A few nurses responded to the situation where there is no physician in a community. Nurses served in other communities that could not support a physician. Some nurses perceived a particular need, such as family crises, child abuse, unmet needs of the aged, or the need for counseling rape victims. In this group there are nurses with a real pioneer spirit, and sometimes missionary zeal. They are aware that they are plowing new ground for nursing. A few have gone into practice to help deprived minorities and the poor. One or two have gone into practice on the assumption that the public does not know what nursing has to offer but that the public needs these services and, ultimately, will pay for them. In a few situations, formally or informally, the community has requested the individual nurse to make her services available.

Equally large numbers have gone into practice because they have been dissatisfied with the kind of nursing they have been able to do within existing agencies, particularly hospitals. They often mention their feelings of powerlessness and dependence under institutional policy and the crippling effects of bureaucratic red tape. They describe the lack of control, autonomy, and authority for their practice. They identify their disillusionment with the lack of patient

contact and with the treatment they receive from directors of nursing, who as administrators are allied with administration and medicine. They are tired of dealing with the threat they pose to directors of nursing and the system as they attempt to practice professional nursing. They feel they are not fairly compensated as skilled clinicians and therapists. They are paralyzed in a health care system that has only a disease focus. While there may be some pioneer-missionary motivation in members of this group, in general they have a greater interest in doing their own thing, developing their own potential, and proving that they personally and as nurses have something worthwhile and special to offer. In this group are some angry people—angry because of the orientation of the health care system, angry because the system could not accommodate them or because the system rejected them.

A few nurses believe that their services have value and that they should receive their fair share of the health care dollar in the same manner as do other professionals in private practice. Imitation of the entrepreneurial, competitive medical model is a very natural route into expanded practice because it is such a traditional, well-known, and financially successful model. Any nurse who is a full-fledged member of a capitalistic society well might ask: "Why shouldn't I have my share of the health care budget?"

Some nurses say that they want to be responsible for and to control their own practice, without saying that this is not possible in practice within agencies. And some report that they want to develop their own potential as nurses and therapists, again without citing the limitations of agency practice for this. A few felt the need to demonstrate that nurses can be successful in private practice and can compete with male therapists.

Other reasons the participants give for going into independent or private practice include the desire to improve the standards of care, encouragement given them by others, invitations by physicians to join them in practice, and the desire to establish a practice base for teaching nursing in a university. Occasionally a nurse identifies the freedom to plan her own working hours or to plan her work around family demands as the reason for setting up a private practice. Continuity of care is an element in the decisions of others.

The women's movement has done a great deal to raise the self-image of nurses. As their egos become stronger they want the power to deliver all they are capable of; they want the status and prestige they have gone without for so long. They want the respect and civil treatment they lacked before they developed an improved profes-

sional self-image. The days of the chronically low nursing self-image are over, and for a multitude of reasons nurses are on their way to demanding and getting what is rightfully theirs.

Occasionally a nurse says she went into practice to test a particular theoretical framework for practice or a particular philosophy of nursing. Most nurses have several reasons for going into independent or private practice, but whatever the reason these people have a sense of manifest destiny, and they communicate excitement and goal-directedness. They are people on the move, and they are in a hurry.

DEFINITION OF PRACTICE

Concern over the lack of a widely accepted definition of nursing is the subject of chapter 8. However, despite the lack of a common definition, there is evidence that nurse practitioners have given considerable thought to theoretical frameworks that guide their practice. One carefully developed framework for independent practice that is based on Rogers' theory has been developed by Kohnke, Zimmern, and Greenidge.[1] Some nurse practitioners indicate that the theory of their specialty is adequate to guide practice. Specific theories used include Gestalt theory and the theories of Freud, Sullivan, Bowen, and Berne. Several nurse practitioners use Henderson's theory to guide practice.[2] Several use the theory of Rogers,[3] one uses Dorothea Orem's theory,[4] and one uses Ingeborg Mauksch's concept of the nursing process in combination with Dorothy Smith's work on assessment.[5,6] Several practitioners indicate that health, illness, or human strength is the focus of their practice. One uses the concept of coping, in combination with the nursing process. Several practitioners indicate that they are developing their theoretical frame of reference as they develop their practice.

IDENTIFICATION OF HEALTH NEEDS

Nurse practitioners have confronted the problem of identifying the health needs they intend to relate to in their practices in a variety of ways. A few have carefully documented a population at risk or a group in need. Some have responded directly to a community's expressed needs and requests for services. Others have

approached health needs by identifying gaps or deficiencies in health care services customarily offered in the society.

The women's movement has identified entire areas of unmet needs of women ranging from growth and development, family planning, awareness training, and female sexuality education to rape crisis and counseling needs. Some nurses have become skilled in these areas and have become recognized leaders in the field.

Nurses involved in health care planning and some of those on university faculties are exploring identification of health needs by examining student experiences, by seeking consumer input, and by asking critical questions for which answers must be found. A few nurses have entered independent practice through the pilot-project route, either alone or in an agency-sponsored project.

SCOPE OF SERVICES

There is no more important policy statement for the nurse practitioner than the one spelling out definitively all the ramifications of a practice. All aspects of practice need to be represented in a statement covering scope of services, skills and limitations, professional relationships with other professionals, definition of nursing and its relationship to medical practice, economics of practice, and laws concerning practice.

A statement on the scope of services will include a description of services the nurse offers. It will say where she will offer them, whether she will follow clients to the hospital, and whether she goes to the homes of clients or works only out of an office or clinic. The statement will list the hours and the days of the week the services are available. The nurse should state explicitly whether the client must have a physician before being accepted. If the nurse accepts clients only from selected geographic areas or only for ambulatory care, this should be made clear. If the nurse will only travel certain distances to clients, this also should be stated. Services the nurse offers should be written conceptually, but in terms clients will understand, such as client needs to be met. Whether the nurse will include the family in the care or will serve people in groups is important. How much physical care the nurse provides, or whether she provides physical care, should also be clarified. If the nurse provides coverage when she is unavailable, she should state who covers, identifying the kind of coverage.

The statement is important in developing client expectations and in preventing frustrations. It is also this statement that can be used in determining whether the nurse is practicing within the law.

One nurse in sole proprietorship who has defined her practice, delineated its scope, and identified her client population is Elaine Nielsen. A description of her practice is included here to amplify the text.

A Nurse in Sole Proprietorship

ELAINE NIELSEN

Elaine Nielsen has been in general practice in family nursing and visiting nursing with all age groups for 18 years. She practices in Beresford, an essentially middle-class community of 7500 people within a 10-mile radius in the southeast corner of South Dakota. She has a one-nurse practice in which she travels 26,000 miles per year seeing 50 to 75 patients per week. In addition, she teaches self-help and Girl Scout classes, attends high school athletic events at the request of school officials, and functions as a volunteer on the ambulance corps. She is the only independent nurse practitioner in private practice in her state.

She went into private practice because the county's elderly physician was ill, and she stayed on after his death. The physician had served the community for 40 years. It seemed to Elaine that the family physician was a key person, very much integrated into the life of the community; so she developed her practice using the family physician as a model for relationships, availability, and involvement. Even though Sioux Falls with its hospitals and specialists is only 35 miles away, there was a tremendous need to have someone in the community who would know the families, who would know what was going on, and above all who would be available. This person plays a key role in the community as a whole, and Elaine thinks this has important implications for nurse practitioners.

She first became involved in helping people find new physicians or specialists they required for their health care. She became a focal figure in helping people make the transition from their long-term family physician to new ones, most of whom were 35 miles away in Sioux Falls. Many people were not able to select a new physician, and they simply told her, "You choose one for me." Most of the new physicians were specialists, and the relationships that individual patients and families had been accustomed to with the family doctor changed drastically.

Beresford is in a four-county area in the southeast corner of the state. Two counties had public health nurses and two did not. One county had been 27 years without a physician or any kind of health care. There was a dire need for all kinds of health and direct nursing care, especially in the schools. Seeing the need was there, Elaine finally went into practice herself. She has had a great deal of support from the physicians 35 miles away, although in the beginning it required a lot of teaching and tolerating and yielded a lot of loneliness.

Elaine operates her business from her home. Ninety percent of her practice is in the homes of her patients. The 10 percent who go to her home are seen at her kitchen table. She would like to have an office, but her experience has been that most of the health problems are focused right in the home, where she sees not only all the family but the home itself. She adds, "You have to get into those medicine chests and see what they've got on hand. You've got to find those sticks of dynamite they have right in the medicine chests that are killing them. They often mix drugs that are not compatible." Elaine uses a four-wheel-drive vehicle and has a snowmobile to get into places in the winter months that a car cannot reach. She has a secretary who takes care of correspondence, filing, keeping records, bookkeeping, and billing.

PAYMENTS

Elaine is usually paid by the patient, but she is also paid by many insurance companies on a fee-for-service basis. Medicare, welfare, and Blue Cross are the only agencies that do not pay Elaine for her services. For all other payers she gives the patient an itemized statement of charges on her letterhead. Private insurance companies pay for her services, but she does not participate in Medicare because Medicare regulations require that the nurse be employed by a public health agency. She refers Medicare patients to the public health nurses in the four-county area if the patients so desire.

The Sioux Falls Medicare office is currently studying the possibility of paying Elaine, but she thinks it may be too time consuming and too expensive to do all the paperwork required by Medicare. She also thinks the paper jungle is ridiculous. She believes that many things could be taken care of on a simpler basis and that the patient would get more and better care for the taxpayer's dollar. The correspondence with Medicare "takes a Philadelphia lawyer to figure out." With the nearest public health nurse 35 miles away, patients in Elaine's community cannot get adequate care under Medicare unless the Medicare program can be revised so that they can pay Elaine. Elaine also thinks that a patient should be able to choose his own nurse, and if she is chosen she is the one who should give the care and be paid. She charges $5 for a 30-minute visit during the hours 9 A.M. to 5 P.M. and $10 per visit after that and on Sundays and holidays. She has a mileage charge for long trips. She tries to keep night and weekend calls to a minimum in order to spend time with her family. She has never taken a vacation since she began her practice. When her husband sees that she is getting too tired, he spirits her out of town for a day, half a day, or an evening to have some time for fun and relaxation. When she is away, patients must contact their physicians if they have problems. She informs physicians she will be away.

In addition to school health and a large acute and chronic physical illness practice, she does a lot of alcoholic counseling. Her work with alcoholics may include drying them out and getting them on their feet. She is pleased with this aspect of her practice, and the patients often ask her to their Alcoholics Anonymous meetings. She does sit in on a meeting once in a while. "It's really been a pleasure to help these people in their problems with alcohol, to get in there and know what they are talking about." She often goes to the jail after the alcoholic has been picked up by the police. She goes in to try to talk the person into accepting care. She has spent entire weekends in jail with some of these people, and this has seemed helpful and useful. She has also been known to put up the bail fee for persons with alcohol problems.

She counsels some disturbed teenagers and works with families who abuse their children. About the only patient problem she does not like to handle is pregnancy, although she does provide sex counseling and marital counseling. She insists that obstetric patients see their physicians. For obvious reasons it is impossible for her to accept suicidal or psychotic patients.

There is no answering service in Beresford, but the municipal power plant answers calls for the police department, the fire department, the ambulance service, and Elaine's practice. The plant has a dispatcher on duty 24 hours per day. Elaine's expense is $16.85 per month to rent her pager, which receives her calls. It provides reliable service, and she has received calls up to 35 miles away. She calls in to find out what the problem is and leaves a message that she will call the patient on her return, or in the event of a crisis or emergency she returns to Beresford immediately.

Elaine has collaborative relationships with the physicians with whom she works. They send her admission and discharge summaries for the patients she refers or those she will follow. When she sends specimens to the clinical laboratory, both she and the physician receive copies of the results. The x-ray center operates on the same basis. When she reviews the data, she consults with the physician as necessary, or when she anticipates that he will want to change medications or treatment. She has established relationships with professors in the medical school at Sioux Falls, and she consults these professors as advisers when clarification or consultation is required. Most of her consultation is with patients' physicians by long-distance telephone.

She has tried for 4 years to get the new medical school in Sioux Falls to consider Beresford as a pilot area for teaching young physicians about working in a community setting where there is no hospital; thus far nothing has materialized. She has urged the directors of the schools of nursing at Sioux Valley Hospital and Augustana College to consider her setting for its possibilities for nursing education, but no one has come to look yet. Several nurses from physicians' offices in Sioux Falls have spent a day at a time with Elaine to get a feel for the community where some of their patients come from.

Elaine has never advertised her service. Her practice has developed by word of mouth. She is active and knows the nursing leadership, and she speaks by invitation before various nursing and nursing school groups. However, in 18 years she has had only one referral from a nurse. She says, "It's very hard for people in our own profession to accept independent nursing practice. They think you're an odd duck or trying to play doctor." She has no problem getting referrals from physicians. At first hospital personnel did not want to spend time providing her with information, but now she feels that hospital personnel have gained respect for and knowledge about what the nurse practitioner does.

She has never had support from the state nurses association, the state league for nursing, or the state board of nursing examiners. She thinks that the nursing practice laws are archaic and that nurses involved in institutionalized nursing still think that "nurses should give baths and back rubs—period." They have rewritten the law, hopefully to allow for expanded nursing practice in a private practice setting, but they did not consult Elaine, their lone practitioner for all these years, on her thoughts about what should be included in the new law. The new law went into effect July 1, 1976.

BACKUP

Elaine has a backup gynecologist who will examine patients she refers. She also has a backup psychiatrist to whom she can refer very depressed patients or patients who appear to need medication. Once she makes a referral, she decides whether she will continue to work with the patient. With psychiatric patients the decision is usually difficult and must be made in light of patient and family history, degree of illness, distance from backup hospital, chances of the patient following medication orders, and her assessment of her own ability to deal with the problem. Several other physicians in various fields have been very helpful in assisting when problems have arisen.

She has part-time legal assistance, but no economic assistance; she has no legal or malpractice problems. She does not have a policy manual, but she does have an advisory board from the community. She has malpractice insurance, $100,000 to $500,000 with the St. Paul Fire and Marine Insurance Company. Her whirlpool, electrocardiograph, walkers, commodes, crutches, and the like are insured separately for both fire and liability. This equipment is worth several thousand dollars.

Early misunderstandings about her practice derived from physicians who thought she was practicing medicine, physicians who discounted the potential of nursing in the home, and many people in the community who thought Elaine cared only for the poor, with her reimbursement to come from the welfare system.

She has hospital privileges and makes hospital rounds once a week for patients in her practice who are hospitalized. She likes to keep a close check on how her patients are doing and what kinds of problems they are having. She talks with the nurses about their problems in nursing and fills the nurses in on what has been going on in the home setting. She believes that this kind of interchange is important in reducing the loneliness and alienation of solo practice. To reduce her own stress she also has conferences with her patients' physicians if problems or difficulties occur. Her working relationships with these physicians are such that if she meets a physician on rounds she can simply announce that she is going to accompany him on rounds or that she wants to go through a patient's chart with the physician.

Before going into practice Elaine worked as a medical nurse, orthopedic nurse, emergency room nurse, and administrator in a small hospital. She did obstetric anesthesia, took histories, and did physical examinations and laboratory work. Still, she has had to study the literature steadily and learn many skills over the years, and as she says, "You can't find all of them in books." She also monitors television nursing courses.

In addition, as part of her practice Elaine lends and rents a variety of equipment including crutches, tractions, intermittent positive-pressure machines, whirlpools, walkers, and hospital beds. Daily she carries with her 50 or more items for use in assessment, care, and emergency intervention, as well as a supply of medications.

Other participants in the conference described the pilot project that launched them into the role of providers of primary care in a nursing clinic:

When we started out we bought a trailer to use as a health center clinic and pulled the trailer out to a selected section of town. We started treating patients; two doctors, two nurses, a lab technician, and a social worker from our staff volunteered. We went out one night a week on Thursday nights. Everything was free. When we first went out there we were seeing about 5 patients a night, but soon it was 15 and then 20. Finally, we were seeing 60 patients after we had already worked a full day. It got to be too much, and so we switched to two evenings a week. Then they built a multipurpose building there with city-county funds, and we moved in there. . . .

The hospital that had been in that area had moved to the other side of town, and there were no health facilities available to these people at all. We decided we would try this as nurse practitioners and open a full-time clinic there. That's how I originally got involved in it. So really my practice was already started by the time I began as a nurse practitioner. We just started a health screening project with senior citizens. They came to us once a month. We selected 200 people who were over 65 years of age and who had not seen a doctor for at least 5 years. Those were the criteria for acceptance, and it wasn't hard to find 200 people. It has grown out of bounds already, and we started screening only 2 months ago. In the past month we have opened another clinic about 5 miles from our first one. There we see all senior citizens who are located in that area. The rest go to the other clinic, so we can take a few more now. We are finding many problems with these people. One fellow hadn't been inside a doctor's office for 42 years, because there hadn't been anything wrong with him. You can imagine what this entailed. He brought his wife with him, and as I started talking with her I looked at her legs. I saw she had pitting edema of her legs. So I said, "How have you been feeling?" She said, "Oh, I've been feeling fine except I've got this little cold and cough." I spent more time with the wife than with the client I was supposed to be looking at. We found that she had a cardiac problem and was totally unaware of it. It should have taken me about 45 minutes for his visit, but it came to 2 hours with the family and only about 10 minutes with him. It happens over and over again. This lady had no idea that a cough could have anything to do with a cardiac problem. To her it was just a chronic cold that she couldn't get rid of. She couldn't relate it. She didn't know that much about health or about her own body needs. Her blood pressure was extremely high; she had the whole works. After we got her to come back and did some lab tests we found that she was a diabetic and had had all of these problems for years without knowing that she had them. She's an example of how complex some problems are.

Another example is the child who comes in with a cold. The first thing I find is the general terrible condition of the child. Usually the child has had no immunizations. At first I thought this was unusual, but it is not unusual at all. I never thought I'd ever find a 10-year-old child who had never had a tetanus shot. But this kind of thing comes up all the time. In a 2-week period 52 percent of my time was spent in talking with people about health problems other than those they primarily came in for. Sometimes I'm sure it is less, but I would say that is the average time spent in helping them to identify their present problems and trying to get them into the health care system.

For a few nurses the identification of health needs to be met has been very general. Where there has been no physician in the community, a nurse may have responded to general awareness or pressure for health care. Where a physician has died, a nurse may have stepped in to partially fill the need. A nurse may have had a strong belief based on personal experience that the emotional needs of cancer patients and their families were not being met or that people who wanted psychotherapy in their homes could not secure these services.

One nurse felt that she had to find out whether she could develop a mental health practice and make it pay. She was told by many people that the city she wanted to incorporate in was overstocked with well-educated people with expertise in the area of psychiatry and that she would not succeed there. She then surveyed four suburbs within 20 miles of the city. She found a suburban area where the only psychiatrists practicing used traditional analytic methods and were getting few referrals. This nurse was criticized for approaching a middle-class population rather than offering her services to those with low incomes, but in fact this middle class did not have available to them short-term, dynamic, and growth-centered services. This nurse has become very successful and does not apologize for offering services to people who needed them.

Another nurse responded directly to health care needs:

We moved to this small community when I was in the last stages of my graduate program. We were new, and this friendly community quickly learned that I was in school and what I was doing. Upon completion of my program people immediately began to say, "Can you do this? Can you do that?" I felt the need to support my teaching with patient contact, so I did move into a comprehensive health care framework as a primary care resource in the community.

Nurses in health care planning are dealing with other kinds of problems:

There's an additional factor in the resistance of some clients to having nurses visit their homes. It imposes on their right to privacy. I've been intrigued with how strongly this has been felt by the working-class population. I'm not talking about particular racial or ethnic groups. I'm talking about ordinary people who say, "Why should I let you into my home? I'll come to you." Then they don't always come, but it's a stronger thing than coming back.

In terms of unmet health care needs, how do we fit into the kind of nonsystem that often occurs in inner cities? How do you do health care when you are only safe if you go in pairs or if you get the person on the corner to go with you? Can we afford this kind of service? What kinds of access do nurses have to urban populations, particularly those living in concentrated poverty areas in cities? Health professionals wall themselves up in agencies, but so much of what needs to be done is right in clients' homes. If we went door to door in large housing projects letting people know we are available and responding to situations presented to us, how would we overcome their suspicion of the public worker who comes around and investigates? Many of the mental health clinics are set up so that they are sitting right across the street from neighborhood housing projects. The workers are literally sitting in their offices watching people becoming more and more disturbed on their balconies across the street. The only time someone intervenes is when the police or firemen are called to go in and drag a person out. How can nurses intervene in this kind of dynamics?

It appears that most nurses bypassed collecting baseline data, doing surveys, or even responding to surveys done by others in identifying health needs they would address. Relating to a population in need or at risk is greatly complicated by the nurse practitioner's expertise, needs, drives, disillusionment with the system, and freedom to move geographically. Medical acceptance or tolerance may have as much to do with the nurse practitioner's selected area of practice as does a population with a health need. In terms of distribution of health care, identification of health needs to be met by potential nurse practitioners may be the essence of success in the future.

IDENTIFICATION OF POTENTIAL CLIENTS

While no detailed data were gathered as a basis for identifying health care needs, there was some idea among nurse practitioners of who their potential clients were. Either they saw obvious needs to which they responded, or a population identified itself as being at risk and asked for service. They did not collect data about numbers of potential clients, but they indicated they had some idea about numbers. For example, a good number of nurses knew that there were large numbers of adults or children or victims needing psychiatric services, and being skilled in some psychiatric treatment modalities, they set out to test or develop their own skills. Occasionally the potential client identified was not the ultimate client. One nurse who set up a family therapy practice was referred only those families no one else could treat successfully. By working very hard she was able to prove she could treat these families, and then she set out to break the pattern of referral so that she could work with a range of families rather than with only the severely maladapted family. Descriptions of two practices will illustrate two common ways of identifying potential clients. Marian Havlovic selected a population whose care is generally agreed by health professionals to be fragmented. Marian thought she had the skills to make these patients' care more comprehensive. Mary Gray was selected by her client group, and she then structured the way she would practice with them.

Part-Time Sole-Proprietor Private Practice

MARY GRAY

I'm Mary Gray, and I represent a rural practice here. My practice is limited, because I have a full-time position on the faculty of the University of Arkansas, School of Nursing, teaching in the Nurse Practitioner Training Program. I deliberately limit the size of my practice because I do not want to dilute the quality of the service I give to people. I am operating within a comprehensive health care framework and being a primary care resource in a community that is 40 miles in any direction from the nearest health service. I commute daily to Little Rock, and several other people who live there also commute daily; but that is not the same thing as having somebody accessible in your daily life to help with health problems. My clients range in age from 2 to 92 years. Most of them are 50 years of age or older.

The community I work in is an ethnic community. It was settled by Italian immigrants at the turn of this century. Most of the people there were raised there and are retiring and dying there. There are few outsiders. We moved there when I was in the last stages of my master's program. Because we were new and they were a very friendly group of people, the entire community knew quickly that I was in school, that I was interested in health care, and that I was doing different kinds of things. They were interested in a social kind of way, but upon completion of my program they immediately began to say, "Well, can you do this for me? Can you do that for us?" I was feeling the need to support my teaching with work with patients.

I am by myself totally. I do not accept patients into my case load without a prior agreement from their physicians to work with me, and the patients have to arrange that. I figured that the last thing I wanted to do was fight with doctors, and if the clients took care of it that would handle the matter. And sure enough it has. In the only situations where a physician did not want to work with me, the client has been ready to change doctors. Whether they change doctors is completely up to them. I lay the alternatives out with them, not for them, and they make their own choices. There have been some changes of physicians. The first time it happened I was a little bit frightened because of the county medical society. But there hasn't been any response from them as yet. I have always let the clients do it and haven't gotten involved in it. Consumers do have the control.

At first I did not charge anything because of my faculty position. As a public employee of the state of Arkansas I am not allowed to have a private practice that generates a second income. But it quickly became obvious that clients would not use me the way I needed to be used to help them. For instance, they would not call me in the middle of the night. So I investigated private duty fees and used them as a guide to charging for my services. Generally I charge $7 per hour for a house call plus 25¢ per mile for travel. I don't always charge that. Sometimes I prorate my fee if it involves only a fraction of an hour.

The physicians are now becoming aware of me, and I have used clients to demonstrate my nursing at nursing meetings and at hearings with Congressman Wilbur Mills. My client responses have been most dramatic. We did one presentation at the annual convention of the Arkansas League for Nursing. A geriatric client went with me, and she made the presentation on what a nurse practitioner is and does. To summarize her very dramatic presentation, she said, "This is the nursing care that allowed my family to survive the wilderness. I don't understand why, after I was 12 years old, I never had access to it. All I know is that I'm grateful and thankful that I have access to it now." For me it authenticated the fact that I'm on the right track. I'm coming back to meet people's need to be well, and that means that I'm not doing to, I'm doing with.

I know that there are no new ideas under the sun, but I'm not so sure nursing is not coming back down the funnel. I think we went up, went out, and are now coming back down. In other professions the leaders are the ones who do the practice. This hasn't been true of nursing. I think this is one of the reasons I'm disenchanted with things like the Council of Family Nurse Practitioners. Full-time educators are insisiting on being certified without maintaining a practice. They should be eliminated in organizations where our leaders should be. And I should be eliminated, too, if I'm not doing practice adequate enough to give me a basis for discussion of patient care. I want to be active in a forum in which I can discuss what I do as a nurse in relation to what patients ask for. I don't want to be where somebody else tells me, "This is what you are supposed to be doing," or "We don't want to do this anymore; you may do it now."

To change the subject, my practice will change as more nurses become community-based and plug into patients' needs. I followed one of my patients to a geriatric program, and in that geriatric program I have created a clinical practice area for students. Now, although I am still the only nurse in private practice in Arkansas, the geriatric program is blossoming into a full-time job for a nurse practitioner. We have done a lot of things in this program.

A Model for Private Practice of Psychiatric Nursing with Patients Who Have Cancer

MARIAN M. HAVLOVIC

Ideally, the delivery of health services should be comprehensive and designed to meet the needs of the total population. But in this country health services are not comprehensive or well distributed for large segments of the population. As the result of maldistribution of health care, other prepared health care personnel have emerged as primary health care providers. The women's movement has given impetus to the acceptance of nurses as primary health care providers. For this role nurses have been prepared in expanded functions and more independent practice. Prevailing societal and professional stereotypes of the nurse, as compared to the physician, present obstacles with which nurses must deal prior to and concurrently with assumption of the independent role necessary for doing primary health care. In addition, for the psychiatric nurse, the prevailing negative community attitude toward psychiatry and the low priorities assigned to emotional needs in the purchase of health care services pose additional obstacles. As a psychiatric nurse prepared at the master's level, I am a primary health care provider in the area of psychiatric nursing for patients with metastatic cancer. This paper deals with the rationale for and development of my private practice.

RATIONALE

Identification of the specific health needs of the population a nurse practitioner intends to meet should be established at the outset. Metastatic cancer has the potential for disruptive effects on virtually every aspect of an individual's life because of the effects of the disease process itself and the individual's response to it. The primary modes of health and social intervention, applied concurrently to foster adequate adjustment to the disease, may include oncolytic therapy, medical supportive care, supportive psychiatric care, physical rehabilitation, vocational counseling, financial support, and legal assistance. The absence of a center with suitable consultants to effect an individualized multidisciplinary treatment approach and the lack of personnel to provide psychiatric service create a major gap in the delivery of care to the population of cancer patients. Any disruptive aspect of an individual's life is to some degree disruptive to the individual's emotional well-being. Through a process of continuous goal-directed verbal exchange a psychiatric nurse can elicit and identify potential problems or problematic situations that may be managed psychotherapeutically or physically or may be appropriately referred. Improvement in the emotional interrelatedness of life conduct and function benefits the individual's psychologic state. The improvement of an individual's outlook enhances his coping ability. In the therapeutic roles of counselor and problem-solving facilitator the psychiatric nurse can be an essential health care provider to the population with cancer.

BACKGROUND

My psychiatric nursing practice began in response to a need for psychiatric care in a population of hematology-oncology clients. My practice evolved over a 5-year period, developing out of the identified needs of this population. There was no one in the situation available or willing to work with metastatic cancer patients. The patients' physician identified his inability to provide continuous, consistent high-quality medical, psychiatric, and other related supportive services in addition to oncologic treatment within the time available. Many of the clients were fearful or had negative perceptions of psychiatry. Their cultural orientation was that an inability to cope with problems within the family indicated a weak character and was a shameful situation.

The private practice ambulatory care facilities utilized are located in the outpatient departments of two metropolitan general hospitals. Two afternoon clinics each week are held in one facility. One evening clinic is held each week to accommodate working clients in the other facility. Approximately 60 percent of the clients have metastatic cancer and are receiving ambulatory cancer chemotherapy. The remaining 40 percent of the clients have benign hematologic disorders requiring periodic medical monitoring. From a psychiatric point of view, these clients constitute an essentially normal population. However, cancer patients are prone to experience an inordinate amount of stress and situational crises that result from their metastatic disease and from their treatment. Many do not possess the psychic stamina essential for coping. Initially, a client is seen by the physician for medical management. The physician refers the patient to me, the psychiatric nurse, for assessment, intervention, and follow-up whenever the patient exhibits emotional problems or difficulty in coping with the disease or its treatment. The consultation I give to physicians is in the form of recommendations for the psychiatric management of the client relevant to his current situational crisis. This may include short-term outpatient management by the psychiatric nurse, suggestions for psychopharmacologic management, or referral for more extensive psychiatric management. I also provide inpatient psychiatric nursing consultation at 14 institutions within the metropolitan area of Chicago. These consultations are requested by the attending physicians. The consultation consists of an assessment of the mental status of the client and a review of the current psychosociomedical situation and the status and efficiency of the coping mechanisms of the client and family. The plan for individual psychiatric management is designed and discussed with the individual who requested the consultation. Evaluation and follow-up of consultation takes place within the context of the outpatient clinic visit. When there is extended hospitalization, this function is assumed by agency staff unless further consultation is requested.

EVALUATION OF PRACTICE

From the outset I identified two major goals for my work: I needed to gain free access to the clients, who had negative views of psychiatry, and I needed to expand the role of the nurse by functioning as a therapist in the delivery of health care to metastatic cancer patients. The goals were to be accomplished using a variety of processes. First, I would perform a function for the client that he identified and accepted as nursing (ie, vital signs). During performance of accepted nursing activities I would engage the client in a guided and goal-directed verbal exchange. Gradually clients would question me, thus providing an opportunity to identify myself as a psychiatric nurse. Once my role was known, the client would usually question the validity of psychiatry in general and the specific function of the psychiatric nurse in his setting. Finally, the client would request the nurse to do psychiatric counseling with him.

Initially the entire metastatic cancer population of the clinic was seen and their vital signs were monitored. Initial engagement and consensual validation were our modes of interaction. Occasionally I provided psychiatric or oncologic nursing consultation to the client's physician.

Gradually the clients began to use the interaction with me to such an extent that there was not time to monitor vital signs. Another nurse was recruited to assume this function. Subsequently I saw all clients briefly during each clinic visit for clinical assessment and did crisis intervention if indicated. The client was also informed of the options of extra sessions or telephone contacts. As an identified case load developed, time precluded my screening the entire population. Consultation regarding the psychopharmacologic management or referral of subsequent cases was effected. I set up with a cotherapist a weekly 2-hour closed-end group therapy session on a trial basis to meet the needs of a greater portion of the population. Although the group met the criteria for success as determined by the cotherapist and clients, the lack of time, space, available staff, and supervision precluded this group from becoming a regular part of the therapeutic program.

As my psychiatric nursing practice continued to evolve, families of clients began to request individual and/or conjoint counseling. These individual and family counseling sessions are requested from the psychiatric nurse directly or by physician referral on a fee-for-service basis. The ongoing evaluation of the practice is accomplished through client feedback and peer review.

The development of such a practice requires an egalitarian relationship between referring individuals and consultant. This nursing role provides the client a service that is not available to the majority of individuals with cancer, and this type of practice represents one model for expanded nursing practice.

PREPARATION FOR PROFESSIONAL ASPECTS OF PRACTICE

One must have realistic expectations if one is to avoid frustration, anger, and disillusionment as one moves into an expanded nursing role, a primary care role, or whatever one calls greater responsibility, authority, and accountability for the health care of a group of clients. To expect understanding, support, and encouragement from one's peers in medicine or nursing or any of the other health professions is to set oneself up for disappointment. As with any change, there is challenge and resistance as all parts of the system shift and adapt. In addition, nurses respond as all alienated people when some members of the group improve their situation. They often disparage and sabotage. One needs to expect to interpret and reinterpret, to debate, to challenge and counterchallenge. Going on the defensive is a losing maneuver.

If one practices alone in either rural or urban situations one needs to prepare for practice by identifying peers with whom to share practice problems and from whom to marshal support when the going is rough. One may want to identify or contract with a consultant in advance. Continuing education resources need to be explored. Isolation and loneliness are nonproductive for both nurse and client.

Commitment to 24-hour availability and responsibility for clients may be difficult to make. It is difficult to adjust to the fact that one's decisions and one's work with a client are to be carried out without the approval or countersignature of a physician or other professional. If one does not plan for relief coverage, one can become exhausted by evening and night calls and after-hours home visits (if these are part of the practice).

Careful exploration of role realignment and thorough review of one's theoretical framework and convictions about care and treatment reduce the number of practice problems for the nurse practitioner. One's practice should be carefully examined in terms of the state's nursing practices act, and insofar as is possible the practice risks one expects to take should be explicit and calculated in terms of outcome. In conjunction with these tasks, nurses need to start developing practice policies. The demands and problems of the clientele will make policy development an evolving activity, but some policy problems should be dealt with in preparation for practice. Nurse practitioners need to consider and decide in advance the rules or policies they will abide by strictly and the ones on which they will compromise.

In terms of public relations, nurses should decide what image they want to project in terms of nursing practice and availability and in terms of relationships with other health professionals. Approaching each image problem separately could present a fragmented picture of the nurse and her practice; one may contradict oneself or present oneself in different ways to different people.

Many nurse practitioners indicate that the greatest priority should be given to nursing expertise. They believe that nurse practitioners should have both depth and scope of clinical experience before taking on their own case load. They believe that knowledge is as important as extensive experience in providing a base for decision-making. Some think that the pioneers will have to be exceptionally good for the nurse practitioner movement to succeed. In conjunction with knowledge and experience, it is important to know one's limitations and to be willing to admit that one does not know. Experienced nurse practitioners emphasize the need for continuing study related to assessment, diagnosis, and drug reactions. Some nurses believe that if the client is not able to benefit from the nurse's skill or if the nurse does not have the skill to work with that client then the system should be open enough for referral of that client to another health worker.

SELLING ONE'S SERVICES TO CLIENTS

Nurses have learned the hard way, and no one believes that a nurse can hang out her shingle and the world will come to her door. Everyone now agrees that planning is the key to developing a practice that will be self-supporting within a reasonable period of time. The kind of planning done by nurse practitioners going into private practice varies, and the priorities they assign the various aspects of planning vary. Some of those who have had the most difficulty in becoming self-supporting stress the importance of having savings or some backup source of support. Most suggest starting practice while carrying a full-time job, or carrying a part-time job until the practice generates enough income.

Very successful nurses in private practice have, as a part of their planning, found ways to be visible for at least a year before they open their practices. They seek a population at risk, they learn the pace and politics of the community, and they develop rapport with local social and health care services and think about how they can articulate and collaborate with what they have to offer. They accept every proffered invitation to speak and to be on committees or to do workshops, they join community special-interest groups, they attend community agency seminars and workshops, and they talk with anyone and everyone about their interest in setting up a practice. While the key word is visibility, it includes the concepts of relationships, interpretation, contribution, and to some extent membership.

It is essential that nurse practitioners not approach the opening of an office with charitable intent. Not only is it unwise personally, but also clients may be suspicious of cheap care and may value it as low as its rates; also, harm may be done to the profession. How can health care planners and economists at the federal level work toward professional-level reimbursment for nurses if nurses feel they are not worth professional fees and they educate clients to undervalue their services? How can nurses sell service and earn a living wage if they don't put a monetary value on the service?

Beyond these basic tasks necessary to sell nursing services, nurses use the routes and mechanisms used by other professionals. At least one partnership was introduced to the public through the local newspaper by the district nurses association. Many nurse practitioners have had featured interviews and pictorial exposure in newspapers, nursing newsletters, or nursing periodicals. Women editors are often good friends of nurses. Women's groups have given support and spread word of various nurses' practices. Nursing registries have referred clients to nurse practitioners. Nurse practitioners have developed publicity materials describing their practices that they circulate to social and health-oriented organizations. Quite a few nurses are listed in the yellow pages of the local telephone directory; some nurses place larger advertisements there to describe their services. One nurse writes a column on nursing and health care for the local newspaper. Where nurses are incorporated on a nonprofit basis, they keep themselves informed of the possible sources of funding for various programs (eg, alcohol programs). One nurse has organized other women health professionals in her area of a large city, and they have developed a mutual referral system that saves considerable public relations time for each individual. Some practitioners subcontract with universities, junior colleges, and hospitals for various kinds of teaching. These activities give them exposure and build trust in their competence.

Almost every professional in practice believes that a satisfied client is the best source of other clients.

These are only a few of the strategies for selling services to clients that nurse practitioners use, but they are the ones that received emphasis at the conference.

Maddy Gerrish is one of the most successful nurse practitioners in terms of the number of people she employs and the size of the clientele she has built in only a few years of practice. She describes her practice as follows:

Expansions: A Pioneering Experience*

MADDY GERRISH

To many people the possibility of a psychiatric nurse owning and directing a private mental health center probably seems even more remote than the possibility of a psychiatric nurse as the primary deliverer of psychological health services. Yet both of these are facts, not ideas. For the past 3½ years I have owned and directed Expansion Inc. and Expansion Foundation Inc. This paper will explore what is involved in such a venture.

From the time of my education and training at the University of Maine, I was taught that a nurse was capable of many things, but it always seemed that whatever the task or duty was it was under the direction or supervision of a physician. The medical model was pervasive. Nurses never gave primary care; nursing was an adjunct, a supplement, functioning at the direction of the physician. Nursing education did not encourage the possibility of a nurse as a private practitioner and certainly did not foster the prospect of owning and directing a mental health center.

When I started doing family therapy in 1963 at Boston State Hospital, there was always criticism of the fact that I was a nurse, and nurses weren't supposed to know how to do therapy. Therapy was the preroga-

**Paper delivered at 1975 meeting of the American Nurses' Association's Council of Advanced Practitioners in Psychiatric Mental Health Nursing, San Diego. Permission of Maddy Gerrish and American Nurses' Association.*

tive of the psychiatrist and sometimes the psychologist. But results were speaking for themselves. Families with whom I did therapy were improving. Still, this was not enough. I was still discounted on many occasions as a competent therapist because I was "just a nurse." Thinking that graduate school would add to my validity as a psychotherapist, I obtained an MS in psychiatric nursing. The education and training I had gained did much to improve my skills in individual, family, and group therapy and also community consultation, but there was never a suggestion that a nurse could work for herself or manage her own practice and perhaps employ others. This kind of thinking was deemed radical and impossible. Yet I believed it was possible. I knew I had skill as a psychotherapist, as do many nurses, but I had not been exposed to the concept of using this skill in a different model than the medical one. I was determined at some point to try. I believed that the public, if given the kind of psychological health services it wants and needs, would come to a nurse; but I had to prove it. Pioneering is always hard, for you have no standard to use for comparison or to use as a guide, and usually there is very little support forthcoming because of the uniqueness of a new endeavor. Fortunately, I have a partner, Eileen Cooney, a psychologist, who was equally interested in establishing a mental health center without the medical model.

Keeping in perspective that we were pioneers and would have to confront many obstacles, we started Expansion Inc. in February 1973 in Bedford, Massachusetts. I was told that Boston was overcrowded with well-educated people with expertise in the field of psychiatry and that I would never ever do anything in Boston. So I thought, "Within 20 minutes outside of Boston there are a lot of people. Maybe that's where I should go." I looked around in the areas of Lexington, Concord, Bedford, and Burlington. The reason I went to Bedford was that exploration showed that there were no psychiatrists there who were using anything but the traditional analytic approach. I found they were getting very few referrals. I was criticized because I was approaching a middle-class population and middle-class people have resources. People said to me, "You should be trying to use your services with lower income clients." What I found was that middle-class people didn't have the services that I was talking about available to them. I didn't have to be apologetic for offering services to people who needed them. Bedford is 20 to 25 minutes from Boston, and we draw from a radius of about 200 miles. We have people who commute from New York, Philadelphia, Washington, Nova Scotia, and Chicago to do therapy with us. There is a real commitment to the kind of growth center that we are.

Expansion is a comprehensive mental health center that focuses on establishing a plan of treatment or growth based on what the individual, couple, family, or group needs and not on making them fit into an existing slot or label. Expansion fosters existing strengths and helps to create options and paths for new strengths to be developed. The emphasis at Expansion is not on pathology, but on growth and every person's right to live life the way he or she chooses. No one can be "cured." There is no magic treatment. No one can be forced to change. The process at Expansion is a shared responsibility where each therapist makes a commitment to every client and every client must make a commitment to herself or himself. There is none of the traditional possessiveness or a closed system structured by therapists in regard to their clients. It is not unusual for a client to see several different therapists during a course of growth and therapy, for we utilize each therapist's skills for the full benefit of every client. This model of sharing provides a very open, free process for change.

Now, a little about the mechanics of the start of Expansion. We estimated that we would need about $2000 capital to start our venture. Simultaneously, we began looking for office space and meeting with a lawyer regarding the choices open to us for doing business legally —whether to form a corporation, a subchapter corporation, or a partnership. We found and rented three offices. We decided on formation of a corporation as the form offering the most potential benefits for our needs. As soon as the legal paperwork was completed we began seeing clients. I had had a part-time private practice for many years and was established with some clients already. The first day we were confronted with the problem of how to record our receipts, but within a week we realized the necessity of setting up a bookkeeping system and acquiring greater business understanding. We went to several accounting firms and were taken aback by the discrimination we encountered. Indirectly the messages we received were these: (1) women don't know how to run a business; (2) we did not have the credentials for such a venture. While several of the firms had handled professional corporations, they had been organizations run by male physicians. We tried to select the firm that had the least negative attitude toward us. Even so, the year was full of difficulties. Finally at the end of our fiscal year we discovered why. They were so convinced that we would not be viable that they were reluctant to give us any time (ie, advice with problems that came up); we were relegated to the least experienced and least knowledgeable employee, etc. We solved the problem by changing accounting firms, first having obtained the names of several women accountants in the area and interviewed them. By this time we were quite clear about how we did and did not want to be treated; we had proved our financial viability quite satisfactorily and could conduct our interviews accordingly.

I must emphasize here the great importance of having excellent help for the legal and business aspects of going into private practice or setting up a mental health center or clinic of any sort. Equally important is cultivating the attitude that you have the ability to understand business and finance and that you can and will do what is necessary to keep adequate, accurate records for your business. It will save countless worries in tax-return preparation and audits.

Another important factor in the beginning stage was becoming known in the community; I spoke about Expansion on every occasion I could find. It was crucial to become known and visible to the public. The public responded. We were giving them what they wanted—individual, couple, family, child, and group psychotherapy that was done with individual planning and assessment. We knew theory and techniques, but we were also able to address ourselves to the practical. Within several months of opening we had to take on two more therapists because the number of clients was increasing so rapidly. This meant, of course, renting more space. Each day presented us with problems and situations we had not experienced before. How to set fees? What about billing? How to do taxes? Do we need a psychiatrist consultant for clients who need medication? What do we do about clients who have health insurance? On and on it went, but the more we experienced the more we learned. We were determined to offer quality psychological services. We did and do. The one factor that got us through all of the beginning hassles was our belief that the Expansion model was viable.

The evolution of Expansion was naturally accompanied by memorable and not so memorable experiences, but I will describe Expansion as it exists currently so that you may see its development. First, the physical space that we rent for Expansion consists of approximately 3800 square feet divided into 17 rooms. There are seven individual therapists' offices, a students' room, a room for acupuncture and massage, a large group room and a small group room, a children's therapy and art room, a viewing room with one-way mirrors into the children's room and small group room, a staff lounge with kitchen, a bathroom with a shower, a staff meditation room, an office for the secretary-bookkeeper with a library wing, and finally a waiting room. We designed the space ourselves, had it executed by an architect, and moved in just 4 months ago. The goal of the design was to provide the most flexibility in use and enough space for many programs to go on simultaneously. The entire space is soundproof.

We see approximately 250 to 300 clients per week. They are referred from a variety of sources, but the majority come from other clients who have been pleased by their therapy and growth experiences at Expansion. At this time there are 16 staff members and consultants involved to varying degrees in programs for varying amounts of time. There are three full-time employees: myself, my partner, and our secretary-bookkeeper. All others are consultants. We are a multidisciplined staff: psychiatric nurses, clinical psychologists, child psychologists, a psychiatrist, an art therapist, an acupuncturist, a muscle therapist, a learning disabilities specialist, a psychic, an astrologer, and a person with a religion and counseling background. The theory of having these people with different backgrounds and skills on our staff is that all too often in our society the helping professions have closed themselves to new theories and approaches to growth and change. They believe in only their own narrow, rigid set and approach. The client is thus faced with only one option in which to learn. We believe that we do not know everything regarding how people grow and change; so we must be constantly aware and open to new routes to growth and awareness. Thus we are exploring what contributions acupuncture, astrology, and the psychic realm can offer as adjuncts to our therapy and to our clients' growth in self-potential.

All staff members receive regular supervision from me, and once a week for 2 hours all staff share together their own work or invite consultants from various disciplines to share with us. While credentials are still important in our society, in staff selection I paid most attention to an individual's own commitment to his or her growth and his or her versatility and openness to an eclectic model. Of particular interest to me, of course, is how psychiatric nurses view this multidisciplined model and work in it. Psychiatric nurses have a great deal of expertise in coordinating various disciplines, but rarely have they used it to their own benefit.

Expansion's sole source of income has been fee for service. Our fee schedule is as follows: $50 for the initial evaluation, $35 per hour for individual, couple, or family therapy, $20 per 3-hour group, $40 to $50 per hour plus travel expenses for consultation and teaching. The evaluation fee is fixed, but all others are negotiable by the therapist and the client. Some of the clients have health insurance, but the majority pay for our services themselves. At this time insurance companies vary greatly in terms of what services, by whom, they will cover. Last year I became licensed as a psychologist in order to keep Expansion under my direction and supervision in the state of Massachusetts and also receive third-party payments. Currently, then, my partner, who is also a licensed psychologist, our M.D. consultant, and I can receive third-party payments. I have not been able to obtain consistent reimbursement as a nurse psychotherapist. While third-party payments are important, and certainly nurses need to be recognized as eligible for these payments, they were not a crucial factor in our becoming viable financially. In order to stay financially viable we try to avoid as much billing as possible. This means that we ask clients to pay for their therapy at the conclusion of each session. This has contributed greatly to making us self-supporting. Many professionals who go into private practice find that after just a few months they are in trouble financially because so much money is tied up in accounts receivable. It is fine to offer good psychotherapy, but if no attention is paid to the financial aspect of the practice, you will soon be out of business. Nurses seem to have great difficulty in grasping the vital importance of this business aspect.

Now, exactly what services do we offer? Let me start with the client evaluation. This is done by me and one of the other therapists at Expansion. It usually lasts 1½ hours, and our assessment is shared with the client or clients as we develop a plan of therapy and growth together. No one is directed into or allowed to choose to go into any form of treatment without an evaluation. Then comes the choice of what modality of therapy will work best. We do not believe that everything works with everyone; thus many different options should be available. We offer family therapy, individual, adult, adolescent, and children's groups, bioenergetics, art therapy, dance therapy, acupuncture, massage and muscle therapy, special tutoring for learning disability, psychodrama, analysis, as well as Gestalt and transactional analysis approaches and techniques. We also conduct all-day marathons for couples, for men only, or for women only, as well as special workshops based on a particular need. We have included these many options because traditional psychotherapy in our society has been done only by a physician offering the same approach to all, which, of course, has limited what the results can be. Also, the public is becoming more sophisticated regarding what is available for help in the psychological realm and is increasing its demands for more options from which to choose.

One final aspect I wish to discuss is Expansion Foundation. This, our nonprofit arm, offers training and education programs and eventually will seek grant support for treatment of those with limited incomes. At various times throughout the year the foundation offers seminars and workshops to the public on such topics as death and dying, parent effectiveness, psychic awareness, etc. We try to offer them at minimal cost so that more people can avail themselves of the opportunity to expand their awareness in a variety of areas. We also have been the field placement for graduate students at Goddard College doing master's work in family therapy and process. In the fall of 1975 and 1976 we offered a multidisciplinary training program for students wanting experience in the broad spectrum of services we offer. Again, should they want to have a formal master's degree, we are working with Goddard College to facilitate this. In conclusion, first let me say that nursing education must revamp curricula and practicums to include more emphasis on the option of private practice for psychiatric nurses. Students must be encouraged to explore whether they have the desire and skill for a venture such as I have described. They must have more opportunities for total responsibility if they are to take such choices. Psychiatric nurses have been afraid to consider options like Expansion because they have not had enough experience with this kind of model. The public is open to services offered by nonmedical models, as witnessed by Expansion, which is going into its fourth year. No longer is it a matter of whether nurses can successfully establish a private practice and a mental health center clinic, it is a matter of when will more nurses take the initiative and risk establishing themselves as primary deliverers of health services in this country. Psychiatric nurses could have the greatest impact on changes in delivery of health services this country has ever seen. But it won't happen without support from each other and from the ANA. We have the expertise, the strength, and the power in numbers to make the changes. We can, as has happened so often with nurses, wait until some other discipline takes over the task and role. We've waited long enough. I have been able to prove to myself what I once speculated was possible. Expansion is not a dream; it is a reality. When more of us can use our abilities in more creative ways we will move in the direction of independence. This independence will establish once and for all that psychiatric nurses are primary deliverers of health care in this country and are crucial to our society's needs.

SELLING ONE'S SERVICES TO OTHER PROFESSIONALS

While nurse practitioners have had a great deal of acceptance by clients, acceptance by other professionals, particularly other nurses, has been a problem for many. For example:

Nurses have been the most unsupportive and unappreciative group. I was asked by a group of public health nurses for a 1-day workshop. I agreed and rented a group room in a centrally located place (my office is in the country). Twelve signed up, but the person making the arrangements did not ask for the fee in advance. Three showed up!

I have yet to receive a referral from a nurse. One psychiatric social worker questioned: "Why am I still getting referrals when you are in practice?" The nurses he was referring to know of my practice.

I found nurses more resistant to my independent role than physicians.

Not one incident but a continuing series of incidents with nurses employed by the local hospital has impressed me with their reluctance to utilize nurses as resources. The nurses I worked with as a CCU nurse and who know me do share cases and problems with me. The new nurses who have arrived on the scene since I worked there are reluctant and sometimes adamantly refuse to share information with me. Very often they choose to ignore my presence, or they greet me with suspicion. I have made several attempts to meet with them in either small or large groups to explain my role, but they have refused to do so.

Although many nurse practitioners have been challenged and required to explain and defend what they do, several nurses describe a more positive experience.

When my preceptorship part was completed, my "doctor associate" and I spent several weeks exploring current area nursing salaries, alternate means for income, office practice expenses, etc. We both spent these weeks feeling quite apprehensive and, at times, uncomfortable, searching for a mutually agreeable reimbursement figure for services. The outcome was, I believe, acceptable to both of us. For the first time in my professional life I felt directly responsible not only for generating income but for keeping most of it for myself. It was a big step in my role change to be directly involved in charging for services, presenting bills to clients, and setting a monetary value on my services.

I have gained respect from the mental health staff (psychiatrists and social workers) in my area because of my work with a multicrisis family they were unable to help.

Most nurses here seem to view the program as another upward trend for nurses as well as women, and they, too, have been supportive.

I have had good relationships with both physicians, nurses, and parents.

When the program was initiated, it was because there was a huge backlog of patients, primarily infants to 3-year-olds, needing "well checkups." The program was needed and wanted by most physicians, and my acceptance by the physicians was no problem.

The physicians have accepted this service more readily than my fellow nurses, I feel. I have received very good support from some of our leading physicians, especially the specialists in their fields. The hospital nurses are very respectful now. I have been in practice 18 years now and have ironed out many bumps in these years. Things are actually going very smoothly at this time.

Several nurses have described problems with physicians: nurse–physician relationships are sometimes a problem. The physician may not understand the functions of a nurse clinician. Thus he may expect too much or too little from her.

A physician recently told me his salary should be three times the nurse practitioner salary. This is based on what his peers make and what the fees are for procedures he performs. I told him the fee schedules are irrational and not based on complexity of tasks. It is also difficult for nurse practitioners to base their fees on those of their peers because there are few such nurses in one's region in similar settings.

I met a psychiatrist in my training workshop who asked about me being his cotherapist in two weekly groups. I charged him my regular hourly fee, $30. He grumbled and waited about 3 months, then hired me for 5 hours a week for about 6 months.

Success in establishing professional relationships with physicians has been mixed. Successful relationships include working with physicians in independent, collaborative, and supportive roles.

Physicians are concerned about the nurses not providing adequate health care without a physician's direct involvement.

Physicians at this institution prefer to label me as a clinician or therapist instead of as a nurse. Neither do they wish to grapple systematically with issues I have raised about the need to differentiate nurse clinicians by levels of skills and preparation for the role.

At the group level, ie, the county and state medical society level, there have been some rumblings and some political pressure exerted in terms of interpretation of the nurse practice act and in terms of revision of the nurse practice act.

There have been occasional local crises, as the following excerpts illustrate:

The state department of health has a large division of primary care with statewide nurse-run clinics. All over the state lots of things are happening. Suddenly, now, we see little legal encounters popping up. They have not hit the nurses yet. For instance, a county health officer lost his job because he refused to supervise a nurse practitioner in a family planning service in a local health department. So he sued to enjoin the state health department and the commissioner of public health to stop providing services where nurses practice medicine. The attorney general threw it out of court. Just like that!

After our office had been open only 6 weeks we were investigated by the state board of medical examiners to see if we were practicing medicine. Local physicians had asked for the investigation after reading a news item about our practice in the paper. Particularly sensitive to the physician readers was the fact that we had a clinical pharmacist working with us. Yet when the local medical society wrote to the state board of nursing to inquire about us, their question was, "Are these nurses practicing nursing according to the law?" Our nursing board's executive director responded that nursing could (and would) regulate its own!

As an aspect of planning, some nurses interested in developing a backup system for referrals have interviewed physicians, hospital administrators, psychologists, and other professionals. But many in this group of nurses indicate that they have never had a referral from a physician or another nurse regardless of the energy expended on the task. One can recognize the threat to medicine if large numbers of nurses have flourishing practices. One can also recognize the typical minority-group alienated behavior of nurses as their peers improve their lot, but this recognition does not make it any easier to build a practice.

Awareness of the importance of planning for change, utilization of change theory, and recognition that innovation is a process would have prevented some of the problems nurse practitioners have had in developing their practices. Timing and allowing time are critical. Mary Alice Hauser analyzed for the conference her experiences in being a change agent. Her experience illustrates the complexity of the task.

Attempts to Develop Alternate Nursing Practice Skills to Improve the Accessibility of Health Care Services for the Elderly*

MARY ALICE HAUSER

PROFESSIONAL NURSE AUTONOMY WITHIN AN EMPLOYING ORGANIZATION

Nurses at the Iowa Veterans Home† in Marshalltown, Iowa, have worked for several years to define and implement a professional model of practice within the employing organization. They believe that nursing services are essential to quality health care, but they are convinced that clients cannot have access to the quality and quantity of nursing services they need unless nurses have control of their practice. Within the Iowa Veterans Home they have been quite successful in defining the scope of their practice and the standards that measure quality of individual and collective practice. By demonstrating their commitment and accountability to clients as individuals and as a group of professionals they have earned the considerable professional autonomy they exercise. They have evidence of improved patient welfare to support their claim to authority.

CONSTRAINTS ON INDEPENDENT PRACTICE

During the process of developing professional autonomy, they encountered two kinds of constraints typical of traditional nursing settings. Some constraints were assumed by nurses, and others were imposed on nurses. Nurses assumed constraints when they lacked professional knowledge and commitment and when they believed there were impediments to their nursing authority even though the impediments were never tested. Assumed constraints included insisting on medical orders for care that was within the scope of nursing practice and should have been deter-

Merideen Maas and Elizabeth Weitzel assisted in the preparation of this paper and contributed considerably to its development.

†The Iowa Veterans Home is a 500-bed health care facility for veterans and their widows. The primary service offered is nursing care, with a variety of other services available. There are three levels of nursing care in which the residents reside: domiciliary care, intermediate care, and extended care. Each of the 21 nurses employed at the home carries a case load of residents with responsibility for planning, implementing, and evaluating their nursing care 24 hours per day, 7 days per week.

mined from the perspective of nursing knowledge and judgment. Examples of such judgments were type and frequency of bathing, level of activity, and prescription of comfort measures. This constraint had some basis in the lack of a theoretical framework of nursing care encompassing these care actions as legitimately nursing. Also lacking was the commitment to serve as advocate for the client and the freedom to take risks. Imposed constraints common to nursing included bureaucratic regulations, unwillingness of other professionals to accept the nurses' authority to order nursing care, and lack of public awareness of nursing's contributions to health care. Examples of imposed constraints were the following: (1) the nursing agency's policy that professional nursing services can be delivered only between the hours of 8:00 A.M. and 4:30 P.M. on weekdays; some of the needs of the clients can be met only after 4:30 P.M.; (2) a belief on the part of many health care professionals, as well as the public, that the client's care is solely the province of the physician, leaving nursing staff no direct access to the client; (3) an institutional policy prohibiting third-party payment for nursing services.

Ironically, the assumed constraints sometimes were institutionalized to become imposed constraints (for example, the traditional rule of public health agencies that the nurse can make only one visit to a client without a physician's order, even though the services needed by the client may clearly be caring rather than curing). Regulations for third-party reimbursement for nursing services now generally follow the model that nursing services must be sanctioned by a physician if payment is to be made. Further, many nursing care activities are not reimbursable at all.

At the Iowa Veterans Home the nurses overcame many of these assumed and imposed constraints and demonstrated that nursing is essential if clients are to receive optimum health care. These achievements were the result of collective action by the nurses who shared a commitment to serve clients. As professionals they defined and controlled their own practice so that clients received optimal benefit. These nurses were not content with the success realized within the agency. They felt an obligation to share their experiences with the nursing profession. Most of them believed that nurses could and should demonstrate nursing as an autonomous professional service in many alternative models. One of their interests was to develop a model of private independent nursing practice in the community.

ATTEMPTS TO DEVELOP A PRIVATE INDEPENDENT PRACTICE

Several years ago four of these nurses began exploring ways to expand the model of practice developed at the Iowa Veterans Home into a community setting. Many of the residents of the home would not need to be institutionalized if they could be helped to meet their nursing needs at home. Many of these needs were of a mental health nature. These nurses received encouragement for an independent nursing practice from the county's board of supervisors, from local, regional, and state public health nursing groups, and from other concerned community leaders. But they encountered constraints: (1) They could not incorporate because of a state law that did not include nurses among those allowed to form professional corporations. (2) They had no access to the existing third-party fee system because they did not meet organizational requirements, because they needed physician's orders for all reimbursable care, and because the reimbursable services included cure functions but not care-oriented functions. The risks appeared to be too great. They were not able to ensure that the practice would receive enough financial support to meet expenses. Although people agreed that the services were needed, no one wanted to pay for them. Because of the constraints and transfer of personnel, this particular endeavor was not pursued further.

A MIXED MODEL IS ATTEMPTED

The same group of four nurses began to conceptualize a model of practice that may be termed a mixed model. The practitioner would be employed part time by the agency and would carry a case load of clients, and part time she would be an independent practitioner in the community.

In the summer of 1975 a proposal was submitted to the Western Interstate Commission for Higher Education for funding as part of a contract for demonstration projects aimed at the distribution of nursing skills and services. A portion of the proposal that was submitted dealt with establishing gerontologic nurse clinicians in two rural communities that have elderly populations exceeding the state average. These nurses would function under the auspices of the Iowa Veterans Home and would provide an outreach activity (1) to make the nursing knowledge of the nursing organization at the Iowa Veterans Home available to people in these two communities, (2) to test the impact of this nursing knowledge and skill on the welfare of these individuals and assess the need for continuation, alteration, and possible expansion of such services, (3) to determine what other resources were needed to postpone or prevent institutionalization, (4) to increase the awareness of nurses, student nurses, consumers, and employers regarding the potential of nursing services in the care of the elderly and chronically ill persons, and (5) to provide educational course experience for registered nurses that would include clinical content relating to gerontologic nursing, as well as exposure to well or worried well elderly. An additional part of this proposal, which was accepted for funding, dealt with the classes for assisting nursing personnel.

Since the time between receipt of the application form for the proposal and its due date was approximately 10 days, exploration of implementation with existing health services was written into the proposal as an activity to be undertaken during the funding period. Contacts were made with the area council on aging and with the area school continuing education department prior to submission of the proposal. Before written confirmation of funding was received, public health nurses in one county inquired of a nurse associated with the project whether she planned to open an office and deliver services. Her affirmative answer set off a chain of events from which we are still attempting to recover.

Essentially, one nurse who had considerable community influence was able to mobilize opposition to the program among public health nurses in several surrounding counties, a few members of the health planning council, one physician, and one county board of supervisors. Letters were written to the editor of the local newspaper. Newspaper articles were written presenting both sides of the issue.

The main objections were that the public health nurses believed they were meeting the need and that the community-based nurses' activities would be a duplication of services. One county board of supervisors felt that the taxpayers would be paying twice for the same service. Another objection on the part of the public health nurses was that the concept of the independent nurse practitioner would destroy the nurse–physician relationship they had "worked so long and so hard to establish." At this point the administration of the Iowa Veterans Home opted not to sign a contract with the Western Interstate Commission for Higher Education because of fear of public disapproval and political repercussions that might jeopardize future programming.

It is important to point out, however, that the nurses received a great deal of support from the communities involved, especially from service clubs. One community offered rent-free office space from which the nurse could operate. The people of the community wrote letters of endorsement to newspapers, county boards of supervisors, and health planning councils. One of the county boards of supervisors recognized the need and value of the service, lending another favorable voice. Thus the end result was a compromise. It was agreed that the educational component should remain as planned, and in addition there would be exploration of a method of delivering nursing services to the aged veterans in the community.

WHAT THE FOUR NURSES LEARNED

The nurses learned several things from their years of attempting to develop an alternative nursing practice model to improve the accessibility of health care services for the elderly in the community. First, they learned of the importance of sound financial backing. Second, they learned that nurses need considerable public and nurse support in the community. The lack of one or the other is likely to result in failure of the independent nursing practice. Financial support can give nurses time to demonstrate services and win the approval of those who oppose them. Community and nurse support can encourage nurses to take the financial risk or endure the hardships of being regularly employed as well as having a private practice. The importance of support from nurse colleagues should be underscored.

The problem of the lack of third-party payment systems for nursing service that is provided directly to clients was highlighted by their experiences. The general lack of knowledge among nurses as to legal and financial aspects of starting an independent nursing practice became most apparent.

Is independent nursing practice a viable, marketable service? In other words, if nurses can overcome assumed constraints, can imposed constraints also be removed to allow private independent practice? Clients are probably the key to this question. Services will have to be demonstrated to clients over a period of time before clients will be willing to pay for services and will demand acceptance of third-party payment. Demonstration of services over a period of time will require financing of some kind. Financing of nurses who desire to open private independent practice should be a subject of considerable priority for the profession.

In addition to building support for their practices and functioning as agents of change for their professional colleagues, some successful practitioners locate the power groups in the community and determine where they stand on the nurse practitioner issues. Then nurses are in a position to seek support through various kinds of relationships with these groups. One power group, of course, is medicine, and one of the first power moves of organized medicine is to make the accusation that the nurse is practicing medicine. It is important not to be entrapped in this issue. It is particularly important not to be defensive. Some nurses suggest going on the offensive. Challengers can be referred to the board of nursing; physicians can be counterchallenged to prove they are not practicing nursing.

Regardless of what nurses do to sell their colleagues on their ideas, they must expect resistance and challenge for a long time to come. It is here that organized nursing could support and intervene.

EVALUATION OF PRACTICE

Peer Review

Nurse practitioners put a high priority on relationships with nurse practitioners and other professionals that make peer review possible and useful.

Nurses concerned about the definition of nursing take the position that each nurse practitioner must be willing to lay out her work with clients for all of her colleagues to hear, to see, to analyze. Every nurse practitioner must in effect say, "What has happened between me and my client I present to you, my peers, as my nursing care." This position demands description of what the nurse says and does in relation to what the client says and does. It requires capturing in words what it is that nurses do. It demands knowledge of the judgments made in the light of what the client presents. It demands knowledge of actions taken and the results of these actions. It demands careful examination and analysis by fellow nurses. And it demands that out of these analyses there must emerge criteria for studying practice and ultimately standards for practice. Out of literal description will emerge conceptualizations of the discipline of nursing, with concepts that modify and clarify theoretical frameworks for nursing practice.

Thus nurses must approach any review of their work with acceptance of the knowledge that they are not presenting the best nursing in the world or the ultimate in patient care. They should feel eager to examine the way they practice, the way they translate their conceptual framework of nursing into practice. Nurse practitioners also need to insist that this is the essence of peer review in nursing and is the only place where standards of nursing can be developed. Some nurse practitioners in this group contend that what are currently called standards of nursing are nothing more than activities that accomplish medical goals. There is some feeling of discouragement that much of the money, energy, and time spent accomplishes just so much more of what nursing has done many times before.

The same nurses who advocate extensive, open, documented

peer review believe that the certification process in nursing is premature and is oriented to medicine at the expense of nursing, as well as lacking in criteria for examining nursing and lacking in knowledge about nursing. These nurses will not associate themselves with peer review because of the focus of the review and because of what they believe to be the medically oriented goals and standards of performance used. There is some interest at the national level in providing a mechanism, at least in psychiatric nursing, for setting up peer review committees to meet the needs of this group of practitioners. Peer review committees would provide opportunities for nurses to share with their colleagues what they are doing and how they are delivering their nursing care.

Another reason that nurses who practice independently give such high priority to developing associations for peer review is their concern about their own effectiveness and growth. When they worked in agencies, association with other nurses provided ample opportunity for all kinds of formal and informal review of practice with colleagues. But when there are no peers close by or even in the same state, regular periodic review of one's practice becomes a critical problem.

Client Feedback

Clients provide some review of practice in terms of the demands they make, the questions they ask, the satisfactions they express, their responses to their care, their continued compliance, and their continuance with the practitioner. One nurse reports as follows on an annual mail survey of clients:

> Following the first year of practice, we polled our clients, using a questionnaire. It covered their satisfaction with the nurse practitioner's services, completeness of calls, follow-up care, patient education, and a comparison of her services with those provided by their physicians. We distributed 150 and had 92 returned. All were positive except for four neutrals and one negative. The one negative had not seen the nurse practitioner. The personal comments were very positive.

One should not underestimate the value of clients' input, but raising the critical questions, making logical analyses, and identifying problem areas cannot be accomplished without input from peers.

Associations for Peer Review

In one larger city several nurse practitioners meet regularly in the evening. They discuss their casework with each other and formulate issues that they then present for discussion with other experts they invite to meet with them. They call this process peer supervision. One cannot help but speculate on how useful the records of this group would be to the profession, if they keep records.

Several nurses who work in various kinds of arrangements with physicians and other professionals hold regular sessions to analyze each other's work. Nurse practitioners associated in this way like the arrangement. They believe they get a better picture of the patient. It provides for a more holistic approach and more comprehensive care for the patient. Nurses find that in time they make better medical diagnoses, and physicians become more adept at making nursing diagnoses. It is very important for those involved in this arrangement to recognize that there is overlap in the areas of assessment and diagnosis. This fact has important implications in joint practice arrangements. But the benefit is that each professional becomes more aware of the total needs of patients. Each professional becomes more capable of making assessments that traditionally have been in the other person's realm of practice. And ultimately patient care improves as the quality of care that each professional can give improves.

There are part-time nurse practitioners who have full-time teaching positions. Some of these teachers work in preceptor roles with students, and in return they have the students review the teacher's work with clients to learn to analyze care, debate care issues, and challenge all aspects of nursing process. Two goals are accomplished at one time as students learn the skills of peer review and teachers have their nursing practice reviewed. Some groups use taped records. In another university setting faculty nurse practitioners present cases to nursing and medical faculty members, pharmacists, social workers, and other resource people.

Some teachers have responded to the needs of graduates of their programs who have had no one to review their work. These graduates prepare records, and faculty members audit them; or where there are large numbers of records they review a random sample. This procedure has limits. Record keeping for this purpose is very time-consuming, especially nurse–client verbal interaction records. Its limitation for the nurse practitioner is that essentially this is an end-point review done after the client's chart is closed. The client is gone. While these are important, nurses should not delude themselves into thinking closed-chart audits have the greatest value. Questions can be raised: "Did you consider this? Why didn't you do that? Were outcomes related to problem solving?" But the nurse does not have the opportunity to revise care or correct errors. Concurrent and periodic reviews and audits have very different values.

One nurse describes the form of peer review that is effective for her:

> There is something that works better than the audit, at least in our situation. We have three nurse practitioners and a physician in our working group. The physician is with one nurse practitioner in his office. I am by myself, and the other nurse practitioner is by herself, except for half a day per week. The doctor comes out and is with her. He is not with me at all. But every Friday we meet together. He presents a case. We each present a case. We select the case we want to present, and we all pick our most difficult one. He picks his most difficult one, too. We present everything we know about the patient—everything that we have identified, social or whatever. If he is presenting, we will say, "OK, what did you do?" He lists everything he did for that patient, everything he said; he tells us what happened. We in turn say, "Why did you do this?" or "Why didn't you do that?" It works far better than a chart audit as far as I am concerned. We just happen to have a physician who will do that with us. He has said many times that he learns so much from what we say to him, just as we learn from what he says to us. It is important to set aside a time for it. It cannot just be a matter of come when it may. When I am away we make up that session. Presenting our cases really keeps us on our toes, a lot more than an audit does. The physician used to come and look at charts. It did not help at all, even when you keep a good record. The big thing that has helped us is that he is on the same level that we are. He's learning from us, and we are learning from him. And we give far better care because of it. It takes a long time to get to the point where you can have that kind of relationship, but I think it is what we need to strive for. You have to grow into this kind of position, no matter who the professional is. The more interaction there is between physicians and nurses, the better assessment and diagnosis nurses do, and the more concerned with the social and rehabilitative aspects of care the physician is.

In one university situation that has an adult nurse practitioner program, peer review for nurse practitioners has been built into the continuing education program offered by the college of nursing.

Some nurse practitioners in isolated settings have tried to set up ways to review practice within regional nursing association meetings. Differences in practice specialties, practice orientations, and academic preparation for practice have made these efforts difficult, although the nurses involved had had some discussion of practice and practice problems. Even without these differences the kinds of relationships required for peer review take time to build.

Whatever arrangements nurses develop for peer review or nursing audit, confidentiality for both client and nurse is important, especially when mailing records and tapes.

One problem in setting up peer review is the wide variation of sophistication in practice, depth of knowledge, and length of practice experience. For some nurse practitioners, finding a baseline level for communication, becoming comfortable with each other, and accepting the differences may take a long time. Finding appropriate resource people in other disciplines may be a difficult task. Finding people who are open, who are not threatened by role overlap, and who can relate as colleagues to nurses is important if nurses are to learn and grow. Nurse practitioners need to accept peer review, recognizing that the process is learned, that skill evolves over time, that becoming comfortable also takes time, and that becoming open to others is one of the most difficult tasks of all.

REFERENCES

1. Kohnke MF, Zimmern A, Greenidge JA: Independent Nurse Practitioner. Garden Grove, Calif, Trainex, 1974
2. Henderson VA: The Nature of Nursing. New York, Macmillan, 1956
3. Rogers ME: Theoretical Basis of Nursing. Philadelphia, Davis, 1970
4. Orem DE: Nursing: Concepts and Practice. New York, McGraw-Hill, 1971
5. Mauksch IA, David M: Prescription for survival. Am J Nurs 72:2189, December 1972
6. Smith DM: A clinical nursing tool. Am J Nurs 68:2384, November 1968

CHAPTER 4

Forms of Association with Other Professionals

For the most part, this chapter provides first-hand reports of various kinds of professional associations. The forms of association covered here are professional relationships as opposed to business and legal structures. There are almost as many forms of association with other professionals and ways of using other professionals as there are nurses in private practice. Nurse practitioners with independent case loads for which they are accountable also structure a variety of working associations. One nurse may have half a dozen different types of associations with other professionals. Some of these associations are basic to the nurse practitioner's concept of practice, and some are complementary or facilitative. Some associations have little or no relationship to the clinical practice, as in the case of a contract with a university for formal teaching, for example. It is apparent that each practitioner has different needs, a different philosophy about practice, and a personal style of practicing and feels comfortable in different kinds of situations. There are also different perspectives on the health care system. A basic necessity in establishing such associations is that the nurse must know when the client is receiving good care and when the client should be cared for by a physician.

A major issue in the private practice of nursing is providing fragmentated versus comprehensive care. Nurses and others concerned about policy in health planning are critical of nurse practitioners who do not seek professional associations that provide comprehensive health services. The whole discipline of psychiatry is under pressure to move psychiatric–mental health services into the mainstream of comprehensive health care. The community mental health movement, with tremendous federal support, effectively perpetuated traditional schisms in health care delivery. Now psychiatry is almost eliminated from recent and proposed legislation. So the mechanism for articulating and integrating these services with the rest of the health care services is yet to be developed and implemented. Psychiatric nurse practitioners going into independent practice are sometimes viewed as perpetuating the worst of the old system, ie, fragmentation of care. But nurses and other professionals continue to increase the private practice ranks of health care entrepeneurs. These groups include sexual counselors, marital counselors, creative divorce counselors, and sensitivity trainers. Nurse practitioners may also practice narrowly in other areas. There are nurses in some parts of the country working only with diabetics, with the mentally retarded, or with the aged. Some of the pros and cons of this issue are explored in the chapter on policy (Chapter 9), but one nurse at the operational level had this to say:

> I'm a generalist, and I think what we're talking about is a philosophical difference. My concern is about fragmentation of care. If I encourage a client to seek a physician's services and I'm not about to provide the input that I feel is needed, or if, let's say, the physician decides to reassess to get another data base or start all over again with the patient, then it is duplication for the patient. I believe in a contractual arrangement, akin to joint practice, with a close relationship with other professionals. We learn each other's language, and we do not duplicate services. The patient does not have to make separate appointments on different days to get total care. He gets it all at the same time. If I don't work closely with physicians, I cannot arrange for total care. It is not a matter of denying the patient total care. It's a matter of not making it available.

HOSPITAL PRIVILEGES

One kind of association that concerns a considerable number of nurses in private practice is hospital admission and visiting privileges. Other nurses want privileges for counsulting in hospitals with physicians who request their services relative to nursing care.

In small towns a few nurses have just gone in and been accepted by nurses and administrators. Usually the patient is under a physician's care, and the nurse goes in to develop nursing care plans, write nursing orders, consult with hospital nurses about a patient's care, or make rounds. In larger hospitals, when nurses wish to write orders and make these orders and their notes part of the clinical record, the problem is more complex. A variety of forms have evolved. Some hospitals allow nurse practitioners to admit patients for skilled nursing care. Some identify the nurse as a member of the nursing staff. Some are identified as being involved in a special project. One is called an hourly private duty nurse, and one is seen as a colleague of physicians. Many of these forms of association are a kind of happening with no formal structure or reciprocal commitments. Others are formal contracts with conditions and privileges made explicit.

Where the hospital administration has questioned the legality of such a professional association, some nurses have been refused hospital privileges. One nurse who was getting no action on her request for privileges described how she got action when one of her clients was admitted:

> I don't know how you would handle hospital privileges, but we have done some interesting things, and it's working out well. My very first patient had to be hospitalized for a nursing problem, not a medical problem. It was in my best interest to be very active in what was going on. I became so active, in fact, that I was really controlling what was going on in nursing.
>
> The physician agreed to the admission and gave medical orders. I then proceeded to call the nursing service administrators and harass them. "I have a patient here. I have a professional responsibility. How are you going to assist me in this?" Every time I went to the hospital (I made sure it was four to six times a day) I called the supervisor to take me to the unit, introduce me to the personnel, and give them instructions that I was to do whatever I wanted to do. It didn't take more than 3 days for them to decide that they would rather have some way of handling the situation other than the way I was handling it. So we developed a nursing staff.
>
> Since then, they have realized that private duty nurses and outside nurses of all kinds ought to be on the nursing staff. Even a nurse who works for a physician, makes rounds with him, and gives verbal or written orders cannot do that anymore just because she is employed by a physician. She has to apply for membership on the nursing staff and be approved by the nursing staff. Staff membership carries with it respon-

sibilities as well as privileges. We have to be involved in and help with inservice education. We have to have our records audited. We have to serve on committees, just as does any member of the nursing staff. But now I can go in there, I am a peer, I am no longer an outsider imposing orders on the nurses. I show up at meetings—staff meetings and care planning meetings. If I have patients, I have input into those meetings. It puts me in a completely different position.

When I first went in there I put myself in the place of the nursing staff. If I were a staff nurse I would feel that no one not on the staff should have any business with a confidential record, and no one not responsible to me should do things to my patient. Also, I would not want to do an outside nurse's work; that would not achieve my professional nursing goals. I intended to carry my nurse practitioner role right into the hospital.

Also, the hospital is liable for everything I do, and this is not fair if I have not proved my credentials. I wanted control of where I would be responsible for the patient. I didn't want to follow a patient into the coronary care unit and have some nurse say I didn't know anything about coronary care. This would not be useful to me in the community. I have privileges in the emergency room, general medical-surgical units, orthopedic unit, regular obstetrics unit, and newborn nursery. But I do not have privileges in coronary care except on a consultant basis related to social support and teaching. I'm just not technically proficient enough to be responsible in that area and should not be allowed to practice there.

I had a patient in the hospital to spend her 3 days for Medicare eligibility prior to nursing home admission. We were going to provide a program of physiotherapy and a speech therapy refresher. When she finally got to the intermediate care facility, she began to have reddened areas over her coccyx. I talked with the nursing staff; I made nursing plans and made visits each morning. None of this was helping; so I was there for a bed bath and taught the aides how to do it. We still didn't get any results, and her skin broke down. So I went five or six times a day again and did skin care and turned her. I proved you could heal it up. So I did bedside care in that institution. Since I follow my patients wherever they go, and since I was giving direct care, I needed privileges there, too.

Other nurses have reported these experiences with hospital privileges:

I sought hospital privileges at two hospitals. I didn't harass them because at first I wasn't aware that I needed privileges. In one hospital I just walked in and the nurse handed me the chart of the patient who needed the nursing care. After I learned this was illegal, I approached nursing administration in two other hospitals. It was involved, and it took at least 6 weeks in each institution. I had to submit my curriculum vitae. I had to talk with nursing administration and explain what it was I could offer; they went through channels to investigate me. They knew their organization, and they decided what would be the most appropriate route.

I was given a staff appointment in one hospital. I was not designated as a nurse practitioner but was identified as "a nurse on a special project." In the other hospital I was a private duty nurse working on an hourly basis. So I did get hospital privileges, and I did it without creating a problem situation after my first error. I did go to staff meetings, and I did inservice education for them. I went to team conferences.

In relation to my patients, I wrote orders on the charts. I just suddenly started to do this without really having permission from the nursing group. They had never worked out what a nurse practitioner is allowed to do in that hospital. I wrote on charts, and I wrote in the progress notes; if I felt a physiotherapy consultation was needed, I ordered that. I also called the dietitian, the physiotherapist, or any other person concerned to discuss what I thought the patient needed. My signature appeared in the record and on the order sheet, but underneath it I wrote our corporate name (this is a corporation of physicians), which I think got it through medical records.

I went into the coronary care unit, into the psychiatric unit, and on the medical-surgical ward. Since we did not have any obstetric patients, I was not involved in that. My realm of practice included the assessment of responses of people to their crises. I went into the coronary care unit and explained what was happening. I was involved in teaching rehabilitation and self-care to the patient, projecting a time frame for convalescence, developing expectations about what was going to happen, identifying job modifications, working out activity modifications, and teaching diet. With hospitalized psychiatric patients I was not the therapist, but more of a liaison person—seeing what was happening with the family and what this individual's response to hospitalization was.

I have struggled bitterly over hospital admission privileges. None of the major hospitals in the metropolitan city area would give me any sort of admission privileges. Now a general hospital several miles north of the city and another one several miles south of the metropolitan area have given me permission for admission. In 3 years we have admitted three people. We meet with people in their homes and build a support system there; so we have little need for hospitalization.

I have never wanted hospital privileges. It never occurred to me to want privileges. Sometimes I'm asked to be a consultant to another health professional, a physician, who is treating a patient in the hospital. I write up my consultation on a consultation sheet like any other consultant. This is highly irregular. Every hospital requires that no one have access to records or write in records unless that person is approved by some group in the institution and is given privileges. Then the physicians call on consultants who have privileges. If the physician knows someone who is especially skilled but who does not have privileges and he wants that person to see his patient, he may have the person come in and see the patient. But that person may not see or write in the record—not legally. Someone called the medical society and said I was doing something I should not be doing, because I had entered as a consultant and used the record. The nurses were agreeable. In fact, a nurse handed me the clinical record, and everything went beautifully until after the fact, when I learned I needed hospital privileges.

I talked with someone who did not appreciate the need for hospital privileges. This was a case of a physician who employed a physician's assistant. The administrators of the hospital thought that since the physician had privileges, and since the physician's assistant was operating on the credentials of the physician who employed and supervised him, they should give privileges to this worker. Since I was a member of a corporation, the hospital administrators took the position that I would be covered by the physician's license. I said: "A doctor can't supervise nursing. I want to be legal." Also, I wanted the recognition.

Despite 2 years of correspondence and interviews with the local hospital administration, I am still not allowed to see patients in my practice who are hospitalized. It was not until I suggested some guidelines and a procedure for nursing staff privileges that I was denied access. At that point the administration refused to talk with me or consider me a separate professional; they will talk only with my physician associate.

As far as arrangements with visiting nurse associations to make referrals, I could call. I could make the referral, but ultimately the corporation name had to appear after my signature. In the case of nursing homes, I found that nursing home people were well indoctrinated to the idea of needing physician signatures and that nursing care cannot be directed by nurses. In one agency I found an administrator who was very interested in the idea and wanted to pursue it. My speciality area happens to be rehabilitation. For example, if we have a stroke patient who has been hospitalized, I follow the patient all the way through. When the patient no longer needs joint physician–nurse care, but only nursing care for adaptation to the disability and self-care instruction, there are occasions when I direct care and the physician withdraws.

NURSE PRACTITIONER AS EMPLOYEE

In a majority of associations involving those using the title nurse practitioner, the form of association is that of employee in a clinic, a physician's office, or a corporate group practice. Sometimes there is a double message in this kind of association. On the one hand, physicians give the message that all are equal members of the primary care team, and in a corporation all are employees of the corporation. The nurse may see as large a case load and may share equally in being on call nights and weekends. On the other hand, when the money is divided, the nurse may get a salary decided by physicians, while the physicians share the profits. Nurses have not generally been successful in buying into or generating membership in the corporation. Sometimes, especially in large structures, the nurse's role as employee is very clear from the beginning, and she accepts the position with this knowledge. In other situations the issue is clouded. The nurse's lack of sophistication in business and the traditional physician–nurse associations get in the way of her thinking through what she is getting into. The employer–employee relationship may also restrict the nurse from making other kinds of association, as the following vignette indicates:

I was involved in a group practice arrangement where I was considered an employee of a corporation. The physicians were considered employees of the corporation also, in that they were also salaried. But the physicians owned the corporation. They owned the shares, and since I did not own shares, my relationship with them was that of employee. At one point I suggested that I resign and enter into a contract with the group to provide services on an independent basis. I was also investigating the possibility of getting into nursing home care, and to do that it would be better not to be a part of a particular group, but rather an independent person contracting with the nursing home. The physicians weren't interested; I had approached it too late. I really should have thought of it much earlier in the planning.

Other nurses describe their experiences:

I've had lots of different forms of association with other professionals. I was in a situation where I was employed by a corporation, and as I look back, what I did there was build the practice. However, when it came time to negotiate for an equitable salary, I was not successful. So I left. That was an important experience, because I reached the point were I said either I would have the same status as physician therapists or I would leave.

At one point we tried to set up a corporation, but in California a physician cannot be in business with a nonphysician. At least that was the rule then. In retrospect we should have explored the possibility of the nurse incorporating apart from the physician group and then having a joint agreement between the corporations. I don't imagine that would have been a problem.

Nurses employed as faculty members in colleges of nursing are being urged to develop a practice base. But many faculty members must make compromises to practice nursing and still stay within the academic setting. Jay Croley, who is highly specialized in Gestalt therapy, conceptualizes a part-time practice job and a part-time teaching job, one separate from the other. She states her position:

In the future I would like to be in a university setting and teach graduate students to use Gestalt, but I'm not willing to be a faculty member, with all the committee work and administrative tasks. It would probably have to be a funded chair. The last contract I had limited me to three specific days a week on campus. The rest of the time I was free to practice. At the contract level I was able to have a lot of input, but at the implementation level it did not work out. They made the same demands on me as on regular faculty members with regular contracts.

Another faculty member tells of being encouraged to practice, but doing so in the university medical center used by the college for student experience. This would limit her control of her practice, her independence, and her freedom to experiment or innovate. In general, faculty members are blamed for not practicing nursing, but structures within which nurses can practice have been slow to develop, and constraints are many.

Some nurse practitioners hope that within the framework of adjunct faculty appointments, preceptor appointments, clinical associate appointments, and clinical professor appointments there will emerge mechanisms that foster clinical practice by faculty members. This would require many nursing faculties to reconceptualize what have most often been courtesy appointments with little meaning and few expectations. One of the problems in seeking this kind of appointment is the lack of uniformity or common meaning for clinical titles in an academic setting. Nurse practitioners will probably have to come to grips with the fact that if a practicing nurse wants a contract with a university, something must be offered in return that will meet certain needs of the university. Currently faculty members are trapped in academic work, and they find it hard to practice part time. Nurses who practice do not want to share the academic busy work; they know the trap and they are wary. It is a problem in the evolution of professional nursing that has not been dealt with in depth. For some time it has been a concern of nursing leaders that faculty members should also practice, but the structures are not there.

One nurse practitioner employee, Karlene Kerfoot, describes some aspects of her practice:

> I work at a mental health center full time with the title of aftercare coordinator. The center is located in a city of approximately 130,000 people. It is a highly industrialized city with a relatively small professional class and middle class within the city. About half of my time is spent in administrative activities. The other half of my time is spent in direct psychotherapy. My practice involves individual and group psychotherapy and sex therapy. My sex therapy case load includes mostly women, but I occasionally do some dual sex therapy with another therapist, a male social worker.
>
> In the clinic I work fairly independently. I do intakes and plan and carry out therapy. I have backup for medications from a psychiatrist. I recommend hospitalization, if necessary, and I can use psychiatrists, psychologists, and social workers as consultants or cotherapists. When I was first employed in the clinic, Title XIX, which is the third-party payer clause for people who are on Aid to Dependent Children in Iowa, did not authorize payment for psychiatric nursing therapy. Blue Cross/Blue Shield was the carrier, and they had to be contacted in Des Moines. After a few meetings they finally agreed to pay for psychotherapy administered by a nurse with a master's degree. In terms of salary, I am the best-paid nurse practitioner in the state.
>
> I also have a part-time private practice as a psychotherapist and sex counselor. I see patients Monday, Tuesday, and Thursday in an office in my home. My practice consists mainly of sex therapy for women, but occasionally I see male patients or couples. My private practice is in Iowa City, a university town. One of the reasons I went into private practice is that I wanted the experience of working with college-age women. I

wanted to do preventive sex counseling with women. I wanted to work specifically with single preorgasmic women before they got into a permanent long-term relationship and before their sexual problems became more difficult to treat.

It was relatively easy to begin private practice. I am fairly well known in eastern Iowa. I was probably the first sex therapist in the area, and I had given many workshops on human sexuality and sex therapy. In addition to a considerable number of television appearances, I have been a frequent lecturer at the nursing and medical schools at the University of Iowa and in health agencies. I started the first human sexuality course at the University of Iowa.

Almost all my referrals have come from physicians and other clients. I have had one referral from a nurse. I had some problems deciding who to accept as clients, because I cannot offer 24-hour-a-day availability. I made a decision not to accept psychotic or suicidal people because I am not available for crisis coverage.

I utilize the services of gynecologists who do gynecologic examinations when needed. I also utilize a psychiatrist if I am working with a disturbed person who needs medication or a person with whom I am having trouble with differential diagnosis. If I determine on initial interview that a person has problems with a major illness, I refer the client to other therapists. For example, a women on initial intake was overtly psychotic during the interview. She had a strong parental history of psychiatric illness that involved several suicides. In a clinic situation I could work with her, but the risks were too great to work with her in my private practice. I referred her to a psychotherapeutic setting with 24-hour-a-day coverage.

I wanted to work with essentially student groups; so I decided on a sliding fee scale of $25 to $10 per hour. Sometimes I question this decision and think, "By God, I'm good and I'll charge everybody $25 an hour." On the other hand, most of the student population could not afford that fee. If I had to support myself in my private practice, I would have to expand, charge full fee, and see clients other than the student population. The way I charge might be considered unfair to other nurses who are starting in private practice, but my case load is so small that I am not a serious threat to any nurse in private practice.

One great disadvantage for me in private practice is that I get a sense of isolation and alienation. I considered going into private practice full time, but I decided I would not unless it was a group practice. I miss, after a really good session or a really bad session, someone to share this with. I would like to say, "What should I have done? Look what I did." I miss the kind of feedback in private practice that I get in the clinic.

Another nurse practitioner, Evelyn Chapman, described her practice and some of its problems in a small group session at the conference. Evelyn went to Big Piney, Wyoming, from Utah 6 months ago as a salaried employee of a Utah-based health care business organization to staff a beautiful new $25,000 clinic built by the county. She was to have a backup physician 2 days every week to take care of medical problems and to give her time away from work.

Big Piney is a town of 570 people in Sublette County, which has a population of 3500. It is located 100 miles south of Jackson and 130 miles northeast of Evanston, Wyoming. It is about halfway between the two. Sublette County has no hospital, essentially no physician, and no laboratory services. The Sublette County Hospital Board provided the impetus for building the clinic and contracted the services of an out-of-state proprietary health service company. The health care service took the overall responsibility of operating the clinic and keeping it solvent as well as provided all necessary supplies and equipment, including x-ray facilities.

Before the Marbleton–Big Piney Clinic (Marbleton is another small town of about 225 people a mile from Big Piney) was built, the physician living in the community was not well and was absent from the area for extended periods. Because of his health the people did not depend on him, and fewer and fewer went to him. Members of a volunteer ambulance corps drove accident victims about 100 miles in one direction or 400 miles in the other to the nearest hospitals. The ambulance attendants had no training; thus there was no way to stabilize patients during the long ride to the hospital. Wyoming is a very conservative state, and there were only eight nurse practitioners working in the state. One of these, a man, was a family nurse practitioner. He worked for the Veterans Administration Hospital. Others worked in Evanston and Laramie. Thus Evelyn became the first family nurse practitioner to work in a rural area. She had immediate and excellent acceptance by the community. They needed and wanted the services she had to offer.

When Evelyn introduced herself to the group at the conference, she began this way: "I'm Evelyn Chapman from Big Piney, Wyoming, and I'm not sure, at the moment, just what I am. For the sake of introductions I'll just say that I'm in sort of a private practice. Certain things have happened in the last 3 weeks that are mind staggering, and I've had some sleepless nights." In the beginning the clinic's arrangement with the health care service worked out fairly well, except for the fact that the physician they sent to the clinic was very young and did not want Evelyn absent from the clinic during his 2-day tour of duty. Within a short while the health service company decided to send him to Big Piney only every other week because they were making so little profit there. Even though he worked in several other clinics, these revenues did not approach his salary of $30,000 per year. Evelyn was seeing four times as many patients as the physician, but still revenues were inadequate.

When this arrangement was only 5½ months old, Evelyn was waiting one day for the physician to arrive to cover the clinic while she was out of town for a 3-day conference. The telephone rang. The call was from the main office of the company. They asked her, "Do you think you could take over and run the clinic?" She said she didn't know, adding, "How could I know?" They replied, "We've got to think about it. We've got a $25,000 salary, clinic space, x-ray equipment, and supplies." She agreed to think about it and left for her conference. The physician came for 1 day and left; so the clinic was uncovered for 2 days, although Evelyn didn't know this. The next week there was a meeting of the Sublette County Hospital Board. There are no medical people on the board. They asked Evelyn to run the clinic, and she said she would try.

She has a contract with a doctor who is willing to cooperate with a nurse practitioner. She also utilizes 8 of the 15 physicians in Jackson for backup. She has a physician who does pathology work and another who reads x-rays for the clinic. So now she is officially the health care person in charge of operating the clinic.

Economics are a problem. The first thing the Hospital Board did was to instruct Evelyn to take the bank account in the clinic's name. Actually she found the account in arrears. All funds are now put in the account of Marbleton–Big Piney Medical Clinic, and all bills go out on the Marbleton–Big Piney bill head. She states her current situation: "I must have $8000 worth of bills and salaries to meet. The county loaned us $2000 to meet outstanding bills right now and to keep up public relations. I really feel sometimes like I'm right, you know, because the people are behind me and they need the services I have to give."

In several quarters the clinic is accepted as a vendor of health care services. Workman's Compensation pays, because they realize that it is better for employers to have emergency care, with x-ray and laboratory work as necessary, than it is to have employees lose 3 to 4 days of work going back and forth to Jackson. Public welfare also pays. Evelyn talked with a hospital administrator and the physicians in Jackson and set up a fee schedule. She has not had a problem collecting these fees except from Medicare, Medicaid, and Blue Cross/Blue Shield. They did find that they were undercharging for x-rays. There are no laboratory services in Wyoming, and there are only two pathologists in the entire state, one of whom does routine laboratory work for $6.50 per test.

In addition to financial problems, Evelyn presented other concerns to her conference group, and Ingeborg Mauksch worked with her on them:

EVELYN: There is a meeting coming up at the Board of Physicians in Cheyenne in January. They want me to come down to explain the role of the nurse practitioner. I just don't feel I have any legal backing at all; I went down to the Board of Nurse's meeting and I helped them make out the rules and regulations we work under—a bunch of copies to show them what we had decided. The deputy secretary of state, the president of the nurse's association in Wyoming, even the Board of Nursing—nobody has had enough experience with the new regulations to know all the answers.

INGEBORG: When I was in Wyoming at your convention last year, I sat in on the board meeting. Wyoming was just changing the Nurse Practice Act. Are you OK according to the new Nurse Practice Act?

EVELYN: The new Nurse Practice Act covers extended nursing role, but it does not say to what depth.

INGEBORG: I wouldn't worry about it. I think one of the problems that nurses engage in much of the time is to ask questions that should not be asked.

EVELYN: What is the nurse supposed to ask?

INGEBORG: You don't need to worry about it. If the doctor does not like what you do?

EVELYN: I have been kind of playing it cool—just going from day to day.

INGEBORG: Yes, but you said just a minute ago that you didn't know if you were covered by law.

EVELYN: I know I'm covered by the extended aspect.

INGEBORG: So I don't know what it is that you're worried about.

EVELYN: Well, because the doctors in Cheyenne have been very adamant about this.

INGEBORG: Let's role-play it.

EVELYN: OK. I'm willing.

INGEBORG: You're the doctor and I'm you. What are you going to do?

EVELYN: First of all, you are going to ask me what I am doing.

INGEBORG: What am I doing? I'm trying to assist people to get the kind of care they need.

EVELYN: Exactly what I tell them!

INGEBORG: And trying to give them the care I am competent to give. I refer them or at least put them through on the telephone to people who can help them more than I can.

EVELYN: That's what I'm doing, but a doctor who was down the other day going through the clinic said, "I am behind what you are doing 100 percent, but I'd like to see something in writing."

INGEBORG: You are not really addressing yourself to the point.

EVELYN: But the point is I'm not covered legally yet by a set of rules and regulations.

INGEBORG: But you're covered by your new Nurse Practice Act, aren't you?

EVELYN: I am afraid of being accused of practicing medicine.

INGEBORG: What are the dynamics of your fear? You are not responding to one thing I'm saying to you. You are moving around trying to find other "what ifs" instead of looking at the law that protects you as a nurse and looking at yourself and your accountability. If the doctor says to you, "How can you dare to do these things?" you can say, "It's not a matter of daring, I am acting within the province of legitimate rights established by legislation in nursing in the state of Wyoming." Then, if he does not like it, he can go to court. He will get no place.

EVELYN: This is what I say to myself every day. Then all of a sudden I'm alone out there. See? I need peer support. There are only three nurses in the whole county.

INGEBORG: You need peer support, but more than peer support you need self-confidence. There are plenty of people there. I would say they are behind you, but they aren't saying that; so you're looking again for a hitch. There is not a light spot in this situation. You can either get out of what you are doing and forget it, or if you are going to do it, look at it positively. You are not doing that.

EVELYN: Oh yes I am. I'm trying to get a look at how you would feel if you were in the same situation.

INGEBORG: If I were in the same situation, I would say, "Will I do this?" I know I am a risk-taker. I am legally covered. I carry good liability insurance, which I pay myself. No institution has to do this for me. That's fine.

EVELYN: That's the way I felt Tuesday, but Wednesday a nurse called. She is a public health nurse. She said, "You know it will never work without a doctor. It's going to fail. You are not going to get the support of the people. People are already talking about it." I don't know what people. I can't see this, because not only am I running the clinic and averaging 20 people a day, but I'm running an EMT for all our research, and I'm also on the board for the elderly. I've only been there 6 months, and I've become established. Everything was going so good!

INGEBORG: What complications do you have with your state board?

EVELYN: I got approval from Cheyenne for the work I do.

INGEBORG: So you're qualified.

EVELYN: I'm qualified.

INGEBORG: You are having a physician write prescriptions?

EVELYN: I write them and he signs them. I have a contract with him.

INGEBORG: Good! So how can you not be covered? Any physician who gives you a signed slip is saying, in essence, "I am supporting you." So what are you worried about? Are there some things you are doing in your practice that you feel a little fuzzy about? It might be in the gray area of maybe you feel you are getting into medicine and that you are not competent?

EVELYN: No, because I feel I'm highly skilled in everything I do. What I'm worried about is all these debts.

INGEBORG: Oh, it's finances.

EVELYN: Yes. I don't know enough about economics.

INGEBORG: Well, have you had anybody come in and say to you: "You've got to do this much, you have got to have this much patient load in order to make ends meet."

EVELYN: No. The county knows nothing about medicine. They don't even know how to order supplies. I even do the purchasing now.

INGEBORG: You need a cost analysis in order to make it viable. Did you as an individual assume the corporate debt?

EVELYN: The clinic had to, according to the lawyer at the board meeting. He said that anything after the 20th of November was our debt. There were debts before this, too. They were local debts, and so the county board said, "Well, we'll have to pay them because of the need for goodwill." We might get $2,000 back from accounts receivable. We took in over $19,000.

INGEBORG: I'm very confused about whether you allowed yourself to be coaxed inappropriately into an economic liability.

EVELYN: I haven't signed anything.

INGEBORG: All right, why are you worried?

EVELYN: I just feel sorry, because I would hate to see this go under for the people in the community. I'm not legally responsible, but my conscience bothers me. I need someone to come in and give me economic advice.

INGEBORG: Before doing that you need to write down what you believe you are able to deliver. Then you need to sit down with whomever the leaders in the community are and say, "This is what I can do; what do you fellows intend to do if you want to continue to grow?" Right now, you impress me as a person who has the problems of the world on your shoulders. It is not your fault.

EVELYN: I know it isn't my fault, because we really did very well. I can't get over it.

INGEBORG: I still do not have a handle on what's really bugging you.

EVELYN: I'm afraid about what the public health nurse said. It's a small community, and you know that in a small community people are very conservative. This nurse feels that we are not going to succeed. I have almost promised the Hospital Board we will succeed.

INGEBORG: So you went out on a limb?

EVELYN: Verbally, yes.

INGEBORG: And that basically is what is bothering you?

EVELYN: Yes. I hate to see it go under. It's a matter of pride. Another thing is that I went in on a salary basis, but then I made a new contract with the company. I was feeling so good. They were going to give me a salary and some of the gross. It seemed to me to be a very good gross. But they got all the gross. But I can always take time off for the labor. It is a shame to get a community's hopes up this high and then just drop it.

INGEBORG: That is the story of the whole world.

EVELYN: But that doesn't make it right.

INGEBORG: No, but I think one of the things we need to face is that we cannot right the world. We need to look at a situation, assess it, and move in where we can be constructive.

EVELYN: I just need comfort and security every so often. I feel like I'm all alone out there.

INGEBORG: You need to let the community take much more of the responsibilty.

EVELYN: This is what I was wondering. I wonder if it is all right if I go ahead and tell the patients about the situation.

INGEBORG: All right with whom?

EVELYN: All right with them, I guess.

INGEBORG: No, I don't think anyone else can decide a thing like that. You need to decide.

EVELYN: I did bring it out in the MT class the other night. I told all of them. We're going to have to pull together, and they're going to have to help me. And I'm going to take Wednesday afternoon off; I'm going to take the weekend off. And they were concerned, saying they felt like I said, "I've got to have a weekend off." I have the answering service in the house.

INGEBORG: It sounds like you hear two messages—a public health nurse says the community is not supporting, but you hear the people saying they are.

EVELYN: Yes. I can't figure out where she got her information. I feel I'm doing a good job.

INGEBORG: Now you're talking!

EVELYN: But the county board says, "You run the clinic. We don't make any decisions. You make all the decisions, but then you're responsible for all your decisions." Well, that doesn't bother me.

INGEBORG: There is still one answer that I'm looking for. There is one aspect of your behavior that, I think, is universally nursing, and I think we ought to emphasize it. We are very devoid of self-worth and of the ability to realistically assess our competence. You need to be able to say, "There's only this much. That's my piece of the pie, and I'm not going to do this." This, I think, is very hard for us to do.

EVELYN: When you become a part of something, it is very painful to see it die.

INGEBORG: I would look at it the other way. It is much more likely to die if you indiscriminately cope in an unrealistic, unconstructive fashion. It is much more likely to survive if you are able to sort out who is to do what and what you can and cannot do, placing the responsibility on the whole community, voluntary or not.

EVELYN: I agree that it has to be the community's responsibility.

INGEBORG: That's the sort of aspect that moves into the other aspect of our caring relationships regarding fees. That is, what about people who say, "How come you are charging the same as a doctor for this? You're only a nurse. I don't think you should charge as much as a doctor." Have any of you come to that?

EVELYN: No. I feel we don't give inferior medical service. We give good nursing care, and we deserve to get paid for it. One thing that happened in the mountain area that had an impact on me is the fact that assistant physicians came in and got $18,000 to $20,000 a year while nurse practitioners were making $12,000 and $13,000. No way would I work for that.

INGEBORG: It sounds to me as if you have accomplished a great deal in a very complex, unstable situation. You need to be sure about that. It is your fears and uncertainties that are much of the problem.

EVELYN: I know that, and it is helpful to talk about them here. I haven't had an opportunity in my isolated work situation.

CONSULTATION FOR SELF OR CLIENT

Nurses have some problems developing forms of association that include consultation and supervision from their peers. To a great extent this is because nurse practitioners cannot identify other nurses who would be helpful. To some degree it may be a matter of minority-group distrust of its members. Nurses talk about their problems in finding someone whose training and personality make them suitable for consultation. Occasionally at national meetings nurses turn to other nurses who have established some reputation as clinicians or teachers. It might be that consultation clinics for nurse practitioners would be a useful component for meetings of organized nursing at state and national levels. A few nurses have been able to provide for regular periodic review of their patient care. A psychiatric nurse practitioner reports:

> I may need consultation, a medical consultation for something that is unclear. For instance, I had a family that was just the most extraordinarily complicated family I had ever seen. There were so many things going on that I wanted a second opinion. I felt the psychiatrist in our community had the training that made him a perfect person to assess that family. So I sent the family to him. I could have said, "I am not going to treat you. I don't know how. I'm going to send you to someone else." But I felt I could treat them. I just wanted my impressions validated. The consultation was for me, and I paid the fee. It was for my benefit, and the costs were not assessed to the clients in any way. I have also used consultation for the client when both the consultant and I worked with the client, and the client paid us both.

Some nurses consider on-call medical consultation on a long-term basis as mandatory to practice. In terms of patient care they believe that if a patient becomes unstable and needs medical care, they should have a built-in backup system. Karlene Kerfoot is one of these:

> Several patients have been referred for sexual dysfunction therapy; I've discovered that they have been depressed and have experienced the drop in libido that accompanies depression. I have been able to refer them for evaluation for medications to a psychiatrist and follow them for supportive therapy. Two clients did not spontaneously remit the sexual dysfunction problems after recovering from the depression, but they responded to sex therapy. If a nurse does not have medical backup, she has two choices: (1) continue to see the patient without benefit of any evaluation that would determine if medication would be of help; (2) terminate the consultation and refer the patient to a psychiatrist who can legally prescribe medication. The first choice is in my opinion not sound, and the second choice precludes the patient and nurse working together. If an egalitarian relationship can be established with a cooperative psychiatrist, this is in my opinion the best solution. If this is not possible, then the nurse is forced to decline patients who need medication.

Simple referral might mean another assessment and double billing for this aspect of care. Built-in consultation also overcomes the hesitancy of a nurse practitioner to call someone on the telephone to verify an assessment, to think through a clinical problem, or to review the patient's program of care. If it proves to be expensive, the nurse may hold back. If it is part of the services covered in a contract with the physician for consultation, the way is clear. This may be covered by putting the consultant, who may be other than a physician, on a retainer; it may be payment for units of time, or it may be for so many hours per year. Several nurses have described consultative activities:

One kind of association I'm interested in (and I just haven't had the opportunity where I've been) is a nurse-to-nurse consultation. I would love to have a diabetic specialist in my community. I don't know how often I have needed that kind of collaboration. I don't know if any of you have done that—work with other nurse specialists.

We have a psychiatric nurse on our faculty. She is also in a group practice with many different kinds of psychiatric people, and she has asked me a couple of times to help her in physical assessment, total assessment for input. She's not interested in learning those fields, but she recognizes the need for understanding the total person before making conclusions.

Some of our patients need to be followed by someone who can do teaching, which is not my specialty. I know that it needs to be done, but I don't do it; a physician is not the right person to do it, although that's the only option at the moment for me. In these communities there have not been enough nurses who were functioning in that way who would accept referrals. In fact, the same thing holds true for dietary services or a dietician. To find a dietician who is not totally hospital-based but who will see people on an outpatient basis is not often easy. I gave one of these some emotional support; now I refer to her. I have in the past worked with a lot of obese patients, and I have them in group therapy; I refer to her for dietary support.

There are nurses who do not see the relevance of medical, psychologic, or social work consultation in their practice:

I have a very unique situation in my practice with patients. My association with other professionals is on the basis of them also being involved with my patients. I see myself as central—the coordinating center for the patient. I do go to other professionals when it is beneficial to the patient. Primarily this has been physicians; I don't accept patients into my case load unless they have a private physician, because I don't intend to generate into medical care. And I don't intend to fight with the physician to be effective for the patient. The patient must work that out before I contract with him for services. The physicians, whose offices are 40 miles from our town, were pleased to get these rural people, most of whom were geriatric, off their backs. They were happy not to be expected to make house calls or to get telephone calls with inadequate data. I call a physician and tell him a patient came to me with a cough. I tell him I examined the patient and present what data I found. I ask, "Is there anything I can do to help you institute what you want to do?" I'm a generalist nurse who is interested in family care and comprehensive health care as an ongoing continual type of management of health and health problems, which includes maintenance. If the client has a medical problem, I refer him to his own physician. It is kind of like the architect who says, "It's time to get the contractor. I've gone about as far as I can go." If a person is going to build a house, he gets himself a contractor and an architect. These two are not the same thing by any means, but they had better work together or they are not going to build a very good house. I see us as individuals who had better work together or we are not going to build very good health. So I'm not really interested in contracting for medical backup. That's the patient's problem. I don't tell the contractor what to do, and the contractor doesn't tell the architect what to do. So I'm not really interested in getting involved in that. Nor am I interested in whether that physician gets paid or not, not really, as far as my nursing is concerned. That's between the patient and the physician. If it is medical, it is their problem. In this sense the patient coordinates his own care in that I don't do it behind the scenes or see him conjointly with another professional or refer him. He already has his own physician. Ultimately I'm working myself out of a job. I expect patients to be independent in attaining good health care, which involves having a primary physician and gaining knowledge in promoting his own health.

I do a lot of consultation in nursing homes. I'm consultant to a large new cancer institute. It is a major step for an institution involved in a physicial operation to have a nurse as a psychiatric consultant.

I have worked on a consultative basis with agencies with a written contract. Much of this has been for teaching. I have taught nurses, ambulance drivers, psychiatric residents, and all kinds of people. This freedom from the bureaucracy lets me look at the needs in a different way, lets me be more creative, and lets me do different and interesting things. I'm freer to experiment. It also leaves me free to say that there are things I can do and be paid for and things I cannot do.

A few nurses employ physicians to do psychotherapy with selected patients; some contract with physicians on an hourly basis to do medical diagnoses or to prescribe medication for patients.

CONTRACTS WITH AGENCIES TO PROVIDE SERVICES

Nurses make contracts for nursing care, workshops, teaching, or other specified services with various groups or community agencies. One nurse contracts to teach semester-length courses at a state college. Another taught a short course at a state college in sex counseling to emergency room nurses. Some nurses contract with the communtiy services units of junior colleges for preretirement planning courses or for retired persons' health workshops. Continuing education units of colleges are another source of contracts for teaching short-term courses and workshops. Some practitioners engage in teaching activities because they enjoy it, others because of their concern with community health, and others to gain community visibility and reach new clients. One nurse described a somewhat different but exciting contract for a workshop:

> There is a small, wealthy residential community of about 5000 people not too far from where we have our office. A representative of the town called and asked if we could teach the townspeople skills about how to deal with loss, how to deal with grieving, dying, and death. We contracted to produce for the town a "Death and Dying Day." They asked for it, and 600 people from the town came together in an open field. We had workshops and sessions about how they could learn skills to help their own families, their neighbors, and their friends when there is a loss. This was something the people of the town felt a need for. There had been a terrible accident, and several teenagers from the town had been killed; six or eight people in the town who were under 30 years of age had died within a year. Then people got together at a town meeting and decided to seek someone who could teach them skills to deal with these catastrophes. They were very receptive to us, because they asked for it.

PARTNERSHIPS AND CORPORATIONS

There are several approaches one can take in looking at a partnership or corporation. The simplest is probably that involving the legal structure for the association of two or more professionals (Chapter 6). At another level one needs to answer to the question,

"How will I find someone to practice with who is interesting, is able to work with me, and is productive?" One psychiatric nurse practitioner answered the question this way:

> I went to a lot of meetings, and I watched people. I also knew exactly to whom I would refer patients and who would refer to me. I spend a lot of time talking with people who might be possibilities. I attend workshops with them. I shop around! It may be self-serving, but I look for people who have something to offer me and who can complement me. I want someone who is a winner, someone who is going to make it. I don't want someone who is going to lean on me all the time. It must be someone who is assertive and self-confident, someone with good clinical skill.
>
> Then, if you both feel you can practice together, you move to another level of consideration. You sit down and you agree on and write down exactly what you both want. You need to have some sophistication in business or good advice to do this. Then you retain a lawyer and have it worked out on a contractual basis. Include such things as how property will be divided if the partnership breaks up, how fees will be set up, who gets the patients who drop in, how you will refer to each other, how money will be managed, and how expenses will be paid.

Another approach for considering practicing with others is in terms of the benefits for client and nurse as compared to solo practice. A partnership or corporation provides ways to share responsibilities for clients. It offers the clients more options for care. If the professionals are in different disciplines, it offers more comprehensive care. For the practitioner it provides a much more holistic view of the patient. It provides intellectual stimulation, continuing education, and peer review. It provides an outlet when one is under stress. It is useful to be able to talk freely when one feels upset or when one is excited. How good it is to be able to say, "You know, these people I'm seeing are driving me crazy!" or "I discovered a fascinating thing today." In group practice, group members provide support and validation. One also gets feedback about oneself. One nurse described her corporate relationship with two other nurse practitioners:

Nursing Consultation, Inc.

LYNN THEUER

I have a 2-year clinical-specialty master's degree in psychiatric–mental health nursing. I had an educational teaching component as well as a nursing clinical specialty in psychiatric nursing. I taught for a number of years and recently quit teaching and went into full-time private practice in a new corporation called Nursing Consultation, Inc. One important factor that influenced this decision was that teaching was at the low end of the salary scale. Physician assistants with no experience were coming into the state at salaries of $18,000 to $20,000 per year, and I knew that my contribution to health care was as great, if not greater, and I believed that I was more skilled in my field.

Nursing Consultation, Inc., is a private practice, specifically in the preventive psychiatric–mental health area and the area of promotion of healing; it also has a maternal–child–family emphasis. One of the members of the corporation is a family nurse practitioner prepared in maternal–child health nursing. And we think that within 3 years our incomes will compare well with the initial salaries of physician assistants in Minnesota.

We are located in a community that is rural, but it does have physicians. It does not have a full-time psychiatrist at the present time. Thus there seemed to be a need in the community for some psychotherapy, because people were being referred 20 to 40 miles away to receive psychiatric services. If they could not afford private care, they would go to the state hospital and get their services there. We had hoped, seeing this need in the community, to set up a service that would be less expensive for these individuals and would be available to them in the home at the time of crisis, since the moment of crisis is when we felt that therapy was most important.

We opened practice on November 1, 1975. The first week we had no clients. The next week we had one. The next week we had three, and now we are up to five (5 weeks later). At this point we have had calls from prospective clients, and several professionals have called about referrals. So we seem to be growing. And in terms of the costs we initially figured, and looking at the projected income, it appears that within 6 months or a year we should be a profitable organization. But we do have to support three people on salaries, and as we expand we also want secretarial services. Office supply costs must also be figured into that.

Where I really feel fortunate is that I have two partners with basically the same background. We have made our service for 24-hour call, and we rotate calls through an answering service. We use the words human services rather than mental health service. The reason we chose the word human was because there is also a community mental health center in town. It does not have a staff of nurses. It does collaborate with the local public health nursing service, which is another service available in the community. There is also a local family and marriage counseling service, again without nurses in the agency.

We wanted to divorce our terminology from all the traditional medical models and make our service an in-between place for people who felt that they needed confidentiality but didn't want to get into the traditional medical bind. We, of course, deal with acute care, and that has made up the bulk of our practice at this time, but one real aim is preventive services. When using the traditional medical approach, clients would assume that there was to be something wrong with the psyche. That's why we chose not to be associated directly with the terms mental health or mental illness.

We plan to expand the scope of reimbursable services to fit our concept of practice. Our first step in this direction has already been taken. Because our service is so new, we are starting with fee for service, but we have printed at the bottom of our brochure that we will accept insurance payments. We take an individual's insurance policy and study it. We point out the lines (portions of the policy) where we think the patient should request payment from the insurance company. For example, if a policy says, "Nursing services and home visits by nurses are covered if ordered by a physician," we encourage the client to take responsibility for obtaining the physician's order for service.

LOOSE WORKING ARRANGEMENTS

Some nurses work on a part-time basis with a cotherapist for group therapy or conjoint therapy with an individual. They may feel that they need to have input from someone with other ways of looking at problems, or they may seek validation for their own observations or their work experience and the specific input that complements their own skills. They work usually with another nurse, a social worker, or a psychologist, with very simple oral agreements about roles and how fees should be divided.

Some nurses also have a list of clergymen to whom they may send clients. Some may have lists of clients with specific problems who may be willing to offer support for clients with similar problems, eg, mothers whose children have died. These volunteer referrals are usually screened so that referral can be made without concern that the person offering support will instead increase a client's guilt. Nurses for whom these collaboration arrangements work speak very highly of their usefulness to clients.

Peer Practitioners' Association

Patty Brandner is a mental health nurse practitioner in practice as a sole proprietor, but she has close consulting/referring relationships with several other professionals that she calls an association. This association does not exist in the legal sense, but only in terms of the interdependent activities among the four members. Each professional operates a practice independent of the others, each maintaining an office within her own home. They operate under one name because it is a way of consolidating an easily identifiable image for the range of services among them. The practice is called Counseling Associates and is located in Dallas, Texas. It includes another mental health nurse therapist, a gerontologist, and a social worker.

Other referral and consulting colleagues include two independent nurse practitioners specializing in adult health who call themselves Nursing Associates, a psychologist attending graduate school, and a social worker specializing in sexuality counseling as Joyce Tepley and Associates. These women professionals have offices and telephone services available in other areas of the city for common use at a small fee.

These associates also contract with various agencies and organizations. They contract with The Women's Center of Dallas as referral counselors, returning 10 percent of the counseling fee to the center. In the last year they have developed a wide network of women's health professionals in their community for the benefit of their clients. This network includes individuals in Planned Parenthood, the VNA, Reproductive Services, several hospitals, the YWCA, the Rape Crisis Center, the District Nurses, and Texas Women's University, as well as several community colleges in the area.

Patty went into independent practice in 1959 because "I wanted sole responsibility for myself, my time, my expertise." At that time she organized and taught childbirth education classes and began to take people in crisis into her home, where her husband and children aided the support process. A graduate degree in mental health nursing increased the scope of her independence. As Patty tells it:

> When I graduated from the program, they told me I'd probably return home and be "just a housewife and mother," that all my education would be wasted as well as the NIMH grant provided by the government. That sort of put me down. Then they told me no one went into independent practice in Texas. What did I think I was going to do? They didn't show much confidence in me, but that increased my determination to go out and show them I could do it.

She feels very strongly about her independence: "I'll leave nursing if, at any time, I am required to be under someone else's supervision, except for a peer reviewer or consultant." She also refuses to supervise anyone else's work, preferring to practice on a peer level with colleagues.

A description of Patty's independent practice is that she provides "*nursing* emotional health-support counseling." Clients who need medications or hospitalization have their own medical resources. Physical health concerns are referred to Nursing Associates, to colleagues in agencies such as Planned Parenthood, or to the client's physician. She refers alcoholics to Alcoholics Anonymous, where she has made contacts, and she supports both the client's and agencies' efforts. She prefers undrugged clients who want to use their intellects to solve their problems in short-term therapy. She determines a client's health and emotional strengths and offers mental health concepts to maintain the client's wellness; follow-up support is offered when the client determines need. Those clients on psychotropic drugs are referred back to the person supplying them for that particular care.

Her particular expertise is in the areas of childbearing, childrearing, sexuality education for youths and adults, rape counseling, crisis care, and women's health. In addition to individual and family counseling, she conducts a monthly mental health support group for women called the "Who Am I?" series.[1,2] People in crisis live within her family for varying periods of time. Her clients are mostly women because of her close association with women's groups.

Dallas is a city of over a million people. In Patty's section of town there are 400,000 people. The women have had little exposure to the women's movement, and they are not greatly liberated. There are powerful forces at work perpetuating the traditional concept of women as being inferior, dependent, and lacking in intellect, with a major emphasis on being attractive to men. According to Patty there are very few women like Lady Bird Johnson in Texas. More nurses fit the female stereotype than the model of a professional person. It is difficult to become a go-getter in this culture. Women professionals have felt inhibited in their health counseling work by these factors operating in the community.

About a year ago Patty sent a general notice to local women health professionals, and nine responded to the proposed meeting. They planned a series of women's health forums, enlisting the aid of many women's organizations and clubs for sponsorship and publicity. The purpose of The Women's Health Coalition, as they called themselves, was severalfold. One aspect was educating women in the community about their health and health resources; another purpose was to see if women health professionals could, as an interdisciplinary body, work together in providing health programs. In addition, women professionals could support each other in their own kinds of practice and learn about each other's services for referral. Not all of the members of the coalition are in full-time private practice, but they all think independently and are interested in women's health concerns.

The Women's Health Coalition decided to offer five health forums covering physical and emotional health, health resources, professional services available in the community, rape, and healthy life styles. Each member of the coalition determined which program she was most interested in providing and then asked other members to work with her. One of the planners, a sociologist and program director of the YWCA, offered the YW facilities for the forums. A nurse (assistant director of Planned Parenthood) planned the forum on women's physical health; Patty and another nurse therapist planned the forum on emotional health for women and included in their program professionals who were not in the coalition. Two forums focused on healthy alternative life styles and were planned by Patty's gerontologist and social worker associates; several community leaders and laywomen joined in the presentations. Another nurse member of the coalition pulled in the Rape Crisis Center and counseling resources for another forum. The participants in the forums, both lay and professional, gained much information for future cooperation and programs of benefit to both groups. One outcome, among many, was the number of self-referrals for services of the participating professionals.

An important benefit for the professionals is that they now have a wide network of resources for referrals and a group of colleagues for consultation and interaction. The isolation that is common among professionals doesn't apply to these women. Working together they can build their individual practices with support from their peers and have more time for practice expansion. This offers a model for other women who are not used to working together and combining professional efforts.

One source of confusion as yet is the complete peer nature of the group—there is no dominant leader and no one telephone number to call. The fact that there are so many disciplines cooperating to educate the community is also unusual.

Patty and her health programs have received excellent news coverage, and one woman editor calls her for resource information whenever she's working on an article about women's health. Patty has published several articles in the nursing literature; she is a member of the western regional group of the American Association of Humanistic Psychology. She was invited to deliver a paper before the International Congress of Social Psychiatry meeting in Athens, Greece, at the first session to include nurses on the program. Her paper was about two experiences with adolescent females receiving crisis care in her home.

Patty's fee schedule is based on a sliding scale; the client decides what the client can afford to pay between the limits of a minimum of $15 and a maximum $35 per full hour of counseling. Patty says that one difficulty with being a nurse therapist is receiving credibility and pay commensurate with that of other professionals, and she recommends acquiring some financial backing with no strings attached to make the practice a feasible choice for nurses.

On the other hand, often Patty likes what she's doing so well that she provides service at no charge. All those who have lived in her home for crisis care have been destitute, and no payment has changed hands. Patty thinks that these experiences add to her knowledge and mutually benefit her and the client. She tells one story about her approach to reimbursement from her early days in practice:

The VNA called me and said, "We've got a couple of elderly women (little old ladies, they called them) who are writing to the governor about our services, and we're getting letters from his office asking why we're not giving these people what they're paying Medicare for." The VNA (they're very defensive) got terribly upset about it. A colleague had suggested they call me. They asked me to go and see the women and see what kind of services they needed. I said I would be glad to do that, and I asked if there was any money in their budget for that. I said I'd make a contract with them, because I call myself a patient advocate, and I felt that was the need here. They first wanted to know if I could help before they found a source for payment. I went and took care of the two women; one of them needed her car and television fixed, but she had been screwed so many times by repairmen that she was afraid to try again. She needed her TV for the times when her arthritis immobilized her, and she needed her car to get her health checkups at a nearby home for the elderly, negating the VNA visits. I got the two women squared away and was working with the VNA nurses on arranging health care when I asked for my pay again. They then said, "Sorry, we couldn't get you in the budget and don't need you anymore anyway; but will you keep working with the women?" I said, "No way." But it broke my heart, because the service was working so well, and I could see a new way independent nurses could work to meet another need in the community. So I told the women that I knew their concern, that they as consumers needed my services, and that they should go right back to writing the governor, and maybe something could be done about the situation.

At the present time she keeps her business expenses to a minimum; her practice pays for her office expenses, car, malpractice insurance, travel expenses, and clothes. Patty's husband's income is used for food and shelter, and she is covered under his medical insurance. One might class Patty as a pioneer rather than an entrepreneur in the health care arena.

Associations required for peer review are described in chapter 3. The informal associations related to acceptance and support are also dealt with in chapter 3. Associations required for professional practice and effective health care are complex, and there are many possibilties. Only a few of the possibilties have been presented here.

REFERENCES

1. Brandner P: Women in groups. Am J Nurs 74:1661, September 1974
2. Brandner P: A matter of identity—new horizon. Nurs Outlook 22:188, March 1974

CHAPTER 5

Scope of Practice: Inclusions and Exclusions

Marvin S. Fish

ON WHOM SHOULD YOU RELY?

Our objectives are to identify the problem, determine the questions that must be explored, consider the interests affected, evaluate the procedures heretofore employed in the pursuit of the solutions, and then decide on a course of conduct that will produce responses and solutions that will achieve the greatest satisfaction of the interests of most of the people involved. Today I would like to consider ten key questions.

The problem is how to determine the areas of activity in which you may legally engage. The first key question: What is permitted as being within your scope of practice? The answer depends on the definition contained in the applicable statute or regulation as approved by the legislature. The second collateral question: What is prohibited as being outside your scope of practice? The answer may be found either in that same legislatively approved definition or in another that defines some other area of practice. If neither is available (as is the case in more than 75 percent of the states), then the third and fourth questions arise: What should be done? What should not be done? Here the analysis must be a comparison between the risks of action versus inaction and benefit versus potential harm. The answer lies in choosing the less dangerous of the inescapable risks.

The fifth question: What can happen if one engages in a prohibited activity? The answer is twofold: if a statute has been violated, the result may be penal sanctions, in the form of a fine or imprisonment, or suspension or revocation of a privilege, in the form of a license. Such statutory violations may also be considered as evidence of improper conduct equivalent to negligent activity, and therefore they may be a basis for liability for damages.

The sixth question follows naturally from the foregoing: Where can I go for an answer? I suggest that you consider two additional subsidiary questions: Does fact create law? Is quality the prime standard for allowability? Fact cannot of itself create law. The fact that everybody does something does not make it proper. Let us suppose that the objective of the entire system of justice and law is to avoid chaos by creating a standard of conduct such that we will all know how to conduct ourselves in the future to minimize the risk of loss to ourselves and to society. And suppose further that such standards of conduct can be created by a variety of individualized, uncontrolled actions by each of us. Should that be the way to create a standard? If it were, each and every individual would stand alone and determine a course of conduct to be followed and the manner in which it is to be carried out. If one should conflict with another, the result would be chaotic and there would be no predictability. The interests of society at large would most likely be ignored or certainly adversely affected unless there were some objective, independent standard or centralized authority that could and would determine which of the conflicting standards should control. In addition, assuming that there was a consensus as to what the standard should be and there was a desire on the part of some individuals or groups of individuals to change that standard, how should that be accomplished? Can it be seriously proposed, and would you accept the proposition, that violations of the agreed-on standard would automatically create exceptions? Suppose, for example, that the speed limit on a particular highway was 55 miles per hour. Suppose, furthermore, that a group of individuals decided to travel that highway at the rate of 75 miles per hour. Should that automatically change the speed limit? In a representative and democratic society, to which we have subscribed and by which we are voluntarily governed through the adoption of the federal and state constitutions, there are other ways to accomplish such changes. It is true, nevertheless, that in some situations in the developmental stages of health professions changes have occurred in the scope of activities in which various personnel have engaged, after which the law has recognized those activities as being within the scope of practice of the particular category of personnel. However, there is a very real danger in relying on such an approach, since there is a risk that the law may not ultimately recognize and give sanction to the new areas of activity for those individuals; and even if it does, it will not act retroactively.

The eighth question: Is quality the prime standard for allowability? This requires a negative answer. The question does not deal with which activity is included or excluded, but rather the manner in which it is carried out, the quality of performance. This cannot be the prime standard, since there is no way of knowing, evaluating, or judging the manner in which a particular activity may be carried out until after the fact. After someone has engaged in a particular activity it is possible to evaluate it, compare it to other standards in the field, and ask whether it was done properly. However, this is retrospective, and it is dangerous. You cannot forsee what the result will be. If the result is that the quality is less than the quality that is in the best interest of society, it is then too late to protect society. Just to test the principle, let us assume that you teach me to perform one relatively simple surgical procedure and that I do it proficiently. Should that automatically allow me to practice that surgical procedure without regard for what the rest of society may say about it? Or if I were to drive my automobile, which is in perfect condition (and I am a highly qualified operator), at the rate of 90 miles per hour, should that rate of speed be the speed limit that applies to me alone? No, quality is not the answer. On occasion we have attempted to assure quality of performance by establishing certain prerequisites and then monitoring or controlling the activity, all to no avail. The failure is not in the process, but in those who have administered the process. The right to change the quality of the services performed is not legally within the domain of those who administer the process of control; that right belongs to groups of individuals acting together in a democratic manner to effect change of the law.

The ninth question: Why do you want to know the scope of your practice? There are at least four reasons. One relates to the law of contracts and deals with agreements between individuals. Since most agreements of employment are verbal rather than written, and yet are perfectly valid under the laws of most jurisdictions, there may be uncertainty as to the activities that a particular nurse has agreed to carry out. If the individual refuses to carry out a particular activity and is discharged, the issue of whether the discharge was wrongful may depend on the definition of the scope of practice as implicitly agreed on by both parties.

A second reason that one would want to know the scope of practice is related to reimbursement for services. When dealing with policies of insurance or with governmental procedures, policies, funding, statutes, and administrative regulations, we find that one must have performed certain services in order to be entitled to receive payment. The nature and extent of the service must be defined so that the practitioner will know when the qualifications for payment have been complied with.

A third reason deals with liability insurance coverage. The practitioner will be covered for professional wrongdoing only when the wrongdoing occurs within the scope of practice as defined in the policy and as allowed by law. The policy of insurance must be read and understood, and you must participate in all ways possible in making certain that the scope of coverage is clearly stated so that you will be certain that it includes your actual scope of practice. If not, and if something goes wrong, you will not have the benefit of that insurance coverage. My present concern is that insurance companies are charging very small premiums to nurses for professional liability coverage with high limits of exposure. In my opinion these premiums will increase considerably in order to reflect the actual scope of risk and exposure on the part of the insurance companies. But until that time, I am concerned that the insurance companies will in many instances claim that the policy did not cover the particular action of the practitioner because she was acting outside her scope of practice, the result of which will be that the nurse will be involved in litigation with her own insurance carrier on the issue of whether the policy covers the particular incident in question. Most likely the primary lawsuit will be defended by the insurance carrier at no cost to the insured practitioner, but the ultimate judgment, if any is rendered, may not be paid by the carrier if the court decides that the activity was not within the agreed risk assumed by the carrier.

The fourth reason for knowing your scope of practice relates to the realm of negligence. Negligence on the part of a professional person while carrying out some professional activity is called malpractice. In this area of law the facts of a particular situation are presented to the court and then compared to the standard of a reasonably prudent professional person acting under the same or similar circumstances. That standard is determined by expert testimony together with written statements, oral statements, records, professional literature, and other data. The jury decides which of the contested facts are true, decides which of the conflicting professional opinions should be followed, applies the chosen facts to the chosen expert opinion, and comes up with the result. If in a particular case the activity in which the practitioner engaged is determined to have been outside her scope of practice, it is quite likely that acting outside the scope of practice will itself be found to be a negligent act, since the reasonably prudent professional practitioner would not have done so.

The tenth question and its corollaries: What attempts have been made to establish guidelines and find answers to these questions? On whom should you rely? What should be done while in search for an answer? In some situations we rely on courts of law; they render decisions on particular controversies that are presented. The problem here is that the court acts in retrospect and deals with acts that often have occurred many years before. Another problem is that the court may not be guided by adequate expertise; thus the ultimate decision, which constitutes a precedent for the future, may be less than satisfactory for practitioners and also for the public. And finally, although the decision may be a precedent for future action, the facts may change in the next case and the result may be different, or the next court may take a new approach to the law. Of course, each state has the right to determine its answers to these questions without regard to what other states are doing, so that the hazard to the profession at large and the individual nurses who may move from one state to another is quite evident.

A second approach has been reliance on the opinions of the attorneys general. The problems here are that such opinions are not equal to pronouncements of law, the various departments may have political pressures exerted on them that affect their ultimate decisions, and, once again, there may not be sufficient agreement for a national standard to result. In many of these situations it is easier for the attorney general to deny a request for an expansion of activities; the denial may not accurately reflect the realities, but it avoids adverse political comment.

Another approach has utilized declarations by professional associations, either acting alone or acting in conjunction with others. Unless the legislature has given such an association or agency the right to make such a declaration and determination, it has no legal effect whatsoever. Once again, in our democratic society the laws that regulate public affairs are determined by representatives of the public in the legislature, which in turn may establish an administrative procedure for carrying into effect the policies set forth in a statute. This is the only way in which this issue can and should be handled. For more than 10 years I have been advocating the creation of a joint commission for the designation and implementation of medical-nursing activities, but it was not until Idaho adopted this approach that the matter aroused public interest and concern. More than a dozen states have since followed this approach. Under these statutes the legislatures have established administrative procedures whereby, in advance, areas of activity can be analyzed and assigned to groups with particular expertise and differing scopes of practice, with the necessary protective prerequisites being established with the advice and consent of the members of the allied professions, as well as with input from representatives of the public, hopefully with a better assurance of control and quality care.

Another collateral benefit from such a procedure is that everyone will know not only what he or she is permitted to do but also what everyone else is supposed to do. Thus each will be able to rely on the competence of others, with the expectation that each will do those tasks assigned to him or her; and if tasks are not done or are improperly done, only the actual delinquent party will be held responsible. This is not the state of the law at present, although I respectfully submit that this is what it should be, and I expect that this will ultimately become a reality.

DISCUSSION

EVELYN BARRITT: Do the formal mechanisms of the courts carry more weight than the informal one of knowing and talking with people in social settings?

MARVIN FISH: Absolutely, they do. Why? The judge making the decision does not want to be criticized by his colleagues. The worst thing a judge can have happen is to have another court reverse him. That is a real put-down, an emotional put-down. The judge wants to be complimented by legal writers, professors, and lawyers. That happens only if he comes to a decision that is in keeping with social purpose and with citations of authority—this case, that statute, this authority, that testimony, this professional literature, that association. If he does not do that, he is just another guy talking through his hat. Certainly in citing precedents and authorities he cannot say, "Now, I spoke to Dean So-and-So one day at a cocktail party, and she said. . . ." He cannot accomplish his objective of being seen as an authority that way. The most effective way to achieve justice is through the formal procedure. . . .

EVELYN BARRITT: But you have just described exactly why women do not get heard in the court system.

MARVIN FISH: That is not true. There is no reason why a women's organization cannot, as an organization, formally write and present its position on an issue to a court that is hearing the issue. You do not have any impediment. You know your expertise and what you have to offer. Chances are that in your arena there will be no other side on an issue. There will be a void, and you will fill it. There is no impediment in being a woman at all. . . .

EVELYN BARRITT: I think we need a long-term process of educating judges and lawyers about issues that we are going to have to deal with and that are going to come up on our cases. If we have contacts through relatives and friends who belong, over a long period of time, to the same organizations as judges and legislators, we can educate them on issues. Then when they are sitting on the bench making decisions they will have information available to them.

MARVIN FISH: In all states the state and county bar associations have meetings and publish magazines. You might write to a bar association to suggest discussing areas of nursing practice that might eventually require their counsel. You would have some input and influence that way. . . .

PARTICIPANT: I do not think you are hearing. We are saying, "Why don't we reverse the process? Why don't the lawyers invite some professional nurses to speak to the bar associations? Why don't you allow us to inform your discipline?" This has been done effectively in Los Angeles.

MARVIN FISH: If you feel there is something you can offer, then make the offer with the assurance that the invitation will be accepted, or at least not rejected ipso facto. Lawyers take excursions all the time into different areas of expertise. They have to know these things. . . .

VIRGINIA WILLIAMS: In Illinois the nursing association has attracted the help of a lot of people who are leaders in their fields and can function as expert witnesses. We have them listed, so that when the need arises they can be available to testify in court, in preliminary hearings, or in other instances when necessary. We have a good communication system.

MARVIN FISH: Lawyers have to be motivated. You need to convince them that they need to learn certain things from nurses. You need to think about how to motivate not only attorneys but also the judges and the legislators who make the laws to listen to your problems and the input you can have. This kind of approach would give you the mechanism of influence you need. . . .

PARTICIPANT: I am wondering about putting into records those things that show your practice very specifically. Is there such a thing as legal protection for that?

MARVIN FISH: No. What we would do is socratically ask you what you think is important for you to know, what you think is important for the next person who sees the record to know, and what you think your accountant, tax adviser, attorney general, or someone taking over the care of this patient would need to know. Write as if you were reading. Protect yourself. Who wants to see it? Why do they want to see it? What do they know? That must be the common denominator. No one can tell you what to include. You need to consider the relevance—medically, legally, and in regard to taxes and accounting accuracy. . . .

NANCY KELLER: We provide copies of everything we get to the clients, since the nurse–client relationship is not protected in its confidentiality. Our lawyer says, "If they have copies of everything, you're limiting the likelihood of a suit, because there is information flow. It's happening, and that's what they want."

SHARON GEDAN: I do a general health assessment that is very simple. For example: "When was your last pap smear? Who is your physician?" I make a contact and tell the physician that we have a mutual patient. I do what I call psychiatric nurse evaluation, which is an identification of presenting problems, with the history, social history, past history, childhood history, and then a nursing care plan. And then, after each session, I do an evaluation of the nursing care plan with changes and brief notes on the patient's progress. I keep those in my office, locked. The patients can read them. I have them available if they want to.

JO VANDER MEER: I would feel very uncomfortable without records. If someone decides to sue you for malpractice, some nurses think that if you don't have records you are safe. But I really feel I should have records.

MARY GRAY: The reason I feel safe is because I think my records are so darn good. I just dare them to prove anything wrong.

JO VANDER MEER: Do you keep your records? I thought I heard you say you don't keep records.

MARY GRAY: My clients have their own records.

JO VANDER MEER: I misunderstood; the patient has the record. Do you also have the records?

MARY GRAY: No, the patient keeps his own records. They are made, and they are well made, but if he is going to bring suit he has to produce the record. So I'm in the same position I would be in if I had them in my office.

JO VANDER MEER: I would be more interested in my having a record, the patient having a record, and having a copy that could be sent when I'm referring, say to physiotherapy or a nursing home. I would certainly want a copy. . . .

PARTICIPANT: What about the location at which records are maintained or kept? Some people have talked about patients keeping records, since they are the patients' records.

MARVIN FISH: There is just one word: proof. In a legal proceeding one is concerned with providing what, in fact, occurred. Everything after that is commentary. . . .

GERTRUDE ISAACS: We say in our organization that the physician delegates the nursing responsibility. Both physician and nurse sign a statement that they will follow this and that the physician will support the nurse if she follows this. The nurse promises to follow the scope of practice. When we moved on into family nursing we went to the state health commissioner and said, "Is there anything within the law that would prohibit us from doing this?" He said, "No, there is nothing in the law that says a physician may not delegate responsibility. . . ."

PARTICIPANT: What about having a primary care license law at the state level, on one hand, and having a law at the federal level that differs from state law?

MARVIN FISH: Opinion. That is all it is. It is not assurance. It is an opinion, and that is all you can get. There are only two results of statutes and regulations. You are dealing with either privilege or license—either of which can be suspended or revoked. Or it could go into the penal sector with fine or imprisonment. That is all you are dealing with. Would the license be suspended or revoked? As a practical matter those things approved by the board of nursing are not disturbed. Why? Because it is the board of nursing that is the agency, in almost every state, that would have to initiate the process of suspending or revoking a license. Although it does not have the authority to say it is OK, it will not disturb you. The other area is that of being subject to fine or imprisonment because of practicing some other profession (eg, medicine) that requires a license you do not have. I know of only two cases that have ever occurred where a nurse was involved like that. These things do not happen as a practical matter. But is it a hazard? Yes, it is. There is a recent article that goes against this statement, but it is wrong. In this instance doctors and nurses set up a program, with decisions made about function in terms of each person's expertise. This interprofessional self-determination of authority is illegal. They are taking a risk. Is it a realistic risk? Are they going to go after them? Probably not. . . .

PARTICIPANT: When there is a federal law that covers you, that takes precedence over a state law, does it not?

MARVIN FISH: In matters of health, safety, morals, and general welfare, the United States Constitution says that only a state can legislate. But the federal government has the power to deal with interstate commerce; so if you are bringing someone across state lines for immoral purposes, then they can even deal with morality. If one is dealing across state lines with narcotics, the federal government can deal with health and safety. And they can control by withholding funds until the Department of Health, Education, and Welfare conditions of participation are met.

CHAPTER 6

Setting Up a Business

ECONOMICS AND THE PROFESSIONAL PRACTICE OF NURSING

The 1 million nurses in this country, as we all know, belong to the largest group of professionals delivering health care. Of all the groups of professionals in the health care system, they have been and remain the least concerned about the politics, the business, and the financing of professional practice. While other groups have consolidated their political and economic positions, nurses have essentially focused on improving the quality and quantity of services available to ever-increasing numbers of people. There has even been a general feeling among nurses that to be concerned about politics and money was in some important way wrong.

Teachers of nursing and practicing nurses do not often think or talk about the monetary value of the nursing care they are teaching or delivering. Are they so immersed in the concept of the weekly or monthly salary that they are not free to say certain care is worth $20 or $100, as the case may be? Although hospital administrators have long complained about the high percentage of the budget that nursing requires, nursing care has not been and is not now itemized on hospital bills. Nor is the cost or value of nursing care put on any list for distribution to patients. When a nurse starts to think about the monetary value of nursing services, it adds a whole new dimension to her work. Nancy Keller reported this experience:

The first time we had a preoperative preparation we had 6 weeks to work with the person in agreeing on what the problems were and to have him sit down with us at the conference table and build his own care plan that went with him to the hospital. We made hospital visits and were in communication with the physician in an advocacy role. We did a home visit and a final office visit on closure of the case. He wanted to pay in advance and said, "How much will it be?" He was the kind of fellow to whom you could say, "We will tell you what it is by how many hours the care will require. Then would you do us the favor of saying what it is worth to you?" His estimate was $3 over what our estimate was for the care package. So he wrote us a check for $500.

The nursing profession, with its low salaries and low employee benefits, has underwritten much of the cost of nursing care and ancillary care for the American people for 100 years. Nursing's approach has been so physician-dominated, so nonactivist, and so compliant that recent demands for improved economic treatment have been labeled self-serving by many of the very professionals who have seen to it that their own political and economic interests have been well served. More nurses are taking the attitude that there must be an end to the profession's essentially unilateral program of do-gooding and there must be increased involvement in the political and economic structure of this country if nursing is to be a viable force in a rapidly changing society. It is the political and financial forces that are in effect legislating health care. Insurance companies, as a case in point, have tremendous power over who gets paid and how much they get paid for health services.

Planning for Private Practice of Nursing

Because of nursing's dedication to care only, nurses who want to go public, open an office, and develop a private practice are often ill-prepared to do so. Idealistic beginning practitioners appear to think that if they give good care God will take care of them. Some are naive to the point that they think going into practice means making the announcement, whereupon automatically the desired number of clients will appear for care. Lack of careful planning, both economic and political, has been responsible for many of the failures of nurses in private practice.

Economically successful nurse practitioners in both private practice and in joint nurse–physician practice stress the importance of planning. Some suggest setting a specified time, say 1 year, for planning. To assure economic viability, some practitioners have built a part-time private practice and a nucleus of satisfied clients while still employed full-time. This provides a source of income until the practice becomes self-supporting. Other nurses who attended the conference had had little success in building a referral system, either before or after going into practice. One nurse who had 850 clients and two offices had had only three referrals from physicians. Nurses have been a poor source of referrals. Some nurses have saved money to set up a practice and to live on until they have become self-supporting. While a few nurse's husbands have supported them until their practices have begun to pay off, few have treated this support as a business investment.

Lead time is an important economic consideration in planning for a self-supporting nursing practice. Lead time refers to that period of time before the practice begins supporting the staff and paying the overhead of operating the practice. Lead time can be short for nurse practitioners who have already established themselves as clinicians in part-time practice or who have become known through workshops or community programs. The nurse practitioners who have been supported by their husbands have not needed to consider lead time. Lead time for others has been long because of low fees related to reluctance to place a value on nursing or inability of clients to pay. Lead time can also be long when third-party payers are involved and there is considerable elapsed time between billing and reimbursement. Some nurses avoid billing whenever possible and ask for payment on receipt of services. This can resolve the problem of having large sums in accounts receivable and little cash on hand. Some nurses have had to seek other sources of funds that will ultimately support their practices, which is very time-consuming for them.

One aspect of planning for supporting oneself when setting up a practice is working out some fairly specific estimates of cash flow. The amount of money available, the operating expenses, the equipment required, and the scale on which the practice is initiated all enter into planning financial structure. For example, whether a nurse intends to buy or rent an office or intends to operate from home makes considerable difference in the flow of cash: no mortgage payments or monthly rent are needed for a home office.

The first step in planning related to cash flow is developing a preopening budget. This requires deciding what is needed to open and operate the practice, as well as how much money the nurse or nurse and other professionals need for living expenses. If a single nurse opening a business requires $1000 per month for rent, food, insurance, automobile, and clothes, if she pays $500 for equipment and $500 for rent for her office for the first and last months, and if she has only $300 per month guaranteed income, she is *not* in practice. She must net $1000 for living expenses and more than $250 to cover office expenses. For example, this means she must see 63 clients who actually pay $20 each within the month if she is merely to live and cover the office rent. If she has only 20 paying clients, she may go to a bank and negotiate a line of credit or a loan to supplement her income until the practice supports her. This is what one must do *before* opening a business. Certified public accountants, bank officers, and lawyers all say that budgeting is the primary thing that people going into business forget. People think that once they open up, the money is simply going to appear. They rob Peter to pay Paul: they start paying personal bills out of the business account, and then when there is not enough money to pay business expenses they mortgage their homes (a personal asset). One way or the other, a high percentage of them are on their way out of business. This is called undercapitalization and is the most common cause of business failure.

Value of Services

Successful practice in any profession requires that the professional and the client agree on the value of the services to be delivered. And there must be enough clients who agree with the professional in order for the practice to succeed. This is the minimum requirement of value. Nursing, with its altruistic, caring history, seems to present more difficulty than other professions, not only in putting a dollar value on care but also in defining or describing the care so that it has economic value to society. Nursing is still viewed by many nurses as an extension or an expansion of medicine. This prevents clarification of nursing as health care with economic value.

Another deterrent to clarification of nursing has come about because of changes in the nursing practice acts where nursing is spelled out using medical terminology and in a medical framework. Both nursing practice acts and nursing organizations refer to dependent functions as if these were nursing functions and not medical functions. The monetary value of dependent medical functions is difficult to ascertain.

At a time in our history when the economics of health care emphasize unit cost, number of people served, and quantity of service provided, the best things that professional nursing offers may be qualitative: the social value of having a baby at home; the social value of being able to stay in one's home as opposed to a nursing home or psychiatric hospital; the value and power of knowing oneself better, understanding one's health needs, and being more self-sufficient in caring for oneself; the social value of having an advocate in the health care system. These values do not fit easily into a unit cost or cost analysis system. We need a million nurses saying, "The service we provide and the gap in health care we fill cannot be filled by any other member of the health team. No one else can meet these needs, because they are nursing needs."

To further complicate the problem of putting nursing on a firm economic base is the fact that nursing is done by so many variously prepared people at so many different levels of competence. The nurse practitioner movement compounds the situation because there are so many kinds of practitioners. There are those whose scope is the whole scope of nursing needs, such as the generalist and the family nurse practitioner. There are those who have been prepared in an area using the medical model, such as the psychiatric–mental health nurse practitioner, and there are those prepared for narrow functioning, such as sex counselors and rape crisis counselors. A few do only treatments and procedures that would fall into the category of technical nursing, if it is the practice of nursing (as opposed to medicine) at all.

Another aspect of the problem of placing a monetary value on nursing services relates to the income of the population served. So often this population is the urban poor, the ghetto or barrio minority, the rural poor, or the aged living on fixed incomes. Nurses find it very difficult to charge what their services are worth, because they know this may deprive clients of an adequate diet or other life-sustaining necessities. The following example illustrates how serious this problem can be, and how serious the consequences for the program described:

A community hospital in one of the New England states was awarded a 5-year NIH grant a few years ago to set up a nurse-operated and -directed primary care health service for a selected segment of the population of the community. It was to be innovative and to become self-supportive in the 5-year period. This was early in the nurse practitioner movement, and the amount of support offered was unusual for the time. The plan was for nurses to do full patient assessment, monitoring, and health counseling.

Referrals would be made from the primary care clinic to other clinics or health care personnel as needed. Two nurses were selected to develop and operate the primary care health service. They had the option of selecting members of a working board to advise and consult with them. They put only physicians on the board, which was their first error, since physicians could not be effective nursing resource people. Their second error was their failure to establish a fee schedule. They found themselves unable to charge a fee for their services, especially with people on low incomes. Within a short time the group lost their funding because it became obvious they could not accomplish the project goals.

Nurses have not learned to say, "If these services are needed and have worth, they should be supported just as other professionals are supported for care provided to those who are unable to pay."

Medicine has had an influence on what some nurses charge, and some physicians have actually stated that the nurse's services are worth one-half, one-third, or one-fifth of the physician's services, depending on the physician and on where he practices, as well as on his relationship with the nurse.

The paucity of third-party payers makes health care delivered by nurses an extra hardship for clients, and this influences nurses' fees. If a patient already pays for Medicare coverage, he is paying twice when he must pay on his own for his nursing care.

Some nurses do not charge for their services because they work for public agencies (eg, a university) and are not allowed to have other income. This situation causes problems of conscience for the client in making demands for care and getting his needs met; it causes problems for the nurse in terms of making the client feel free to ask for services and in terms of satisfaction in work, since receiving money for work is part of the satisfaction for most people. No contract exists between client and professional unless the terms of exchange for services rendered are explicit.

Medical schools set up structures and procedures for dealing with the fees for services rendered by physicians' employees. While part of the fee is used for administration, the physician often receives a percentage of the fee added to his income or a percentage of the fee to be used for research or teaching overhead or both. If nurses in the academic setting are to assume clinical leadership functions, this area of economics needs consideration.

Lucille Kinlein explains her original low fee schedule this way:

In the beginning I had to be sure that what I was offering the public as nursing was deemed to be valuable to the identification of nursing.

Service was one of the goals that I had when I started the practice. I had to be sure that monetary considerations were not affecting the reasons that people were coming back to me. If people had thought that my nursing service was worth the fee but could not afford to pay the fee again and again, and so did not return, I would not have known whether they did not come back because my nursing care was not useful or because they could not afford the fee. To obviate that occurrence, at least in the beginning, I set my fees very low.

Several nurses have told how their fees were set too low because in thinking through their preoperating budget they failed to take into account how much time, work, and communication with physicians and other health professionals were going to be required. Also, they did not take into account the time and cost involved in travel, particularly in rural areas.

We need to look at what we are doing when we do not charge what is necessary. A lot of things happen to people who receive services for which they feel they are not being charged enough. A whole dynamic is set up in terms of what a nurse is effectively saying to a client who is charged one dollar when he thinks he should be charged five dollars. What is one saying? One can be saying a variety of things: "I don't think my services are good enough." "I still have to take care of your financial, medical, nursing, and emotional needs." "My self-concept is such that I have to underwrite the cost of health care." The economics of the professional practice of nursing are complex, and overcoming the widespread low self-concept the profession has developed during the last few decades is not the least of our problems.

We need, at some point, to take a stand and say, "There are federal and state agencies that supplement all kinds of health services. Why are not nursing fees supplemented as well as physicians' fees?"

The protocols from the small group meetings that provided the major content of the preceding section reflect contributions by Sarah Archer, Maddy Gerrish, Mary Gray, Gertrude Isaacs, Nancy Keller, Lucille Kinlein, and Lawrence Subrin.

STARTING A NURSING BUSINESS

Lawrence I. Subrin

The dictionary defines the noun nurse as "a person who is skilled or trained in caring for the sick or infirm. . . ." The verb to nurse, therefore, means to do what a nurse does: take care of the sick or infirm. I see this definition taking on a new dimension in today's world. Nurses not only take care of those who are ill or weak, they play a larger role in the health maintenance area and in monitoring and consulting services. I see nurses stepping away from traditional roles in hospital settings to a more community-oriented or business-oriented setting. My eyes have been opened in this area through my professional relationship with Nursing Care and Consultation, Ltd. This represented something very new to me. For those of you who have decided to go public or who are contemplating going public with your nursing practice, I would like to share some observations. Although leaving the safe, secure life of the nurse-employee to go out into the cold business world entails added responsibilities, there are greater opportunities to earn money commensurate with the additional risks. We ought to consider what being your own boss means. The risks include opening yourself up to a great deal of liability in the legal sense, as opposed to the financial sense. The financial liabilities are that you commit yourself to a certain number of orders and you commit a certain amount of money. If you order or buy something and do not pay for it, then you have a financial liability.

What individual *really* wants to work for somebody else when there's an opportunity to do it all yourself, to make your own decisions, to make a house call in your particular case or not to make a house call if you so decide, to accept or not accept a client? Answering this question is critical, even primary, to the decision to go into business for oneself. This must be one of the reasons why you decide to leave the protective atmosphere of a hospital where you work from eight to five, or at least have steady hours. There you do not have to worry about hiring and firing. You do not have to worry about the benefits or about paying the bills at the end of the month. All those problems are taken care of. On the other hand, if you accept these responsibilities inherent in an individual practice, the remuneration you receive generally offsets the risks after a period of time. No one who opens up a business is going to be a millionaire overnight, but in the long run, taking the intangibles and the tangibles together, there is no more satisfying way of leading a quality life. You perform a service for the public, and assurance of the quality of that service, besides the increased income, makes for a good life.

If you sit down and carefully map the necessary steps into the private sector of business and plan your time and moves, you will receive the rewards as a natural by-product of your efforts. One of the most rewarding parts of practice is the rapport with clients.

Every client of mine is different, and every patient of yours will be different. If you do not set up a creative program for them, and if you do not set up a creative program for your own internal accounting to evaluate whether you are succeeding from a service standpoint, and from the end result (Are the dollars there?), then you really have not accomplished anything.

Although you are all in a service-oriented profession, you have to remember that you are in it to make money. To be your own boss you have to be comfortable in being the boss and be able to put a monetary value on your services. Determining the charges for services you perform is not an easy decision, but it is a very important one. You have to define your area of service, and then you have to define what those services are worth. How much do you want to charge for them? Because there is a lack of competition (ie, you cannot go down the street as I can and find out what the local CPA firms are charging), you alone have to make the determination. If you are just starting, that is very important. And after a period of time (6 months or 1 year) you ought to reevaluate your fee structure. People often undersell themselves. If you do, you may never get your fees up to what you think you are worth. Start off the very first day charging a fair fee that you are comfortable with. It is better to lose a patient or client before they get involved with you than to have an account that will never be collected. A dissatisfied client can create all kinds of havoc, because very often everybody knows what everybody else is doing. Bad news goes around quickly. Dissatisfied clients are bad news to any professional. You need to write fees down in some kind of brochure that you can make available to prospective patients or clients. This is always subject to review and is very important. At the end of the year you may be satisfied as can be, but you may have lost $10,000. You have begun a service, but you will not be around long enough to complete it. If you have made the decision to go out on your own, you need to understand that money is going to be the natural by-product. Otherwise, do not give up the safety of a hospital or a nursing home.

When you are your own boss you must develop your own clientele, and you must support yourself and your business while you do this. You may think that when you open an office people will be knocking your door down. It rarely happens. You cannot overtly solicit. This means that the bulk of referrals must come from previous connections with clients or professionals who can refer clients to you. After a period of time your own clients will become your best referrals for new clients.

Forms of Businesses

Nursing as a business can develop in any number of ways. For example, you can have a sole proprietorship, which simply means you are the only owner of an unincorporated business. A husband and wife (defined by the government as one person) also can have a sole proprietorship. Or if there are two or more individuals who are owners (not necessarily equally) of the business, they can go into a partnership situation, sharing the associated responsibilities and liabilities.

There is a variation of the partnership form that is known as a limited partnership. It has all the trappings of a regular partnership, except that the limited partners, as opposed to general partners, have limited financial liability.

Probably one of the most interesting business vehicles utilized is the corporation, whether it be a profit or nonprofit entity. It has rules and regulations specified by law. Even though you may own all the stock in the corporation, you are governed by certain general regulations set up by the corporate laws in that state. The corporation often becomes more restrictive than other business forms, but obviously, since there are so many corporations around, they must also have advantages. These advantages include limited liability; also, corporations are allowed more fringe benefits. Corporations can offer better pension plans or profit-sharing plans. An individual in a partnership can have tax deferral or retirement plans, but at this time, generally speaking, these plans are not equal to corporate plans. A corporation may have a sick-pay inclusion. Corporations may have what they call medical reimbursement. This means a corporate entity may pay your medical bills as an employee and then get the deduction for those medical bills. It is not income to you, even though you benefit by it. You cannot do that in a partnership because you take if off on your own tax return, but on your own tax return the federal government limits most of these deductions to approximately 4 percent. All business entities have some commonalities. For example, they all must have some kind of bookkeeping system. They must have some way of saying how much was taken in, how much was spent, who owes what, and who is owed. The larger the organization, the more activity, the more people involved, the more sophisticated is the accounting system. Either the sole proprietorship or the partnership can evolve into a corporation. Most clients, for various reasons, tend to have either a sole proprietorship or a partnership. The advantages of one or the other are that the guidelines or the parameters of these entities are less restricted. You can do more things in the sole proprietorship and partnership without having to document. Also, the legal fees of incorporating are often high, and cost very often is a serious consideration to a new business. The least expensive form is the sole proprietorship, and this fact is a real consideration. The corporation does involve a form of limited liability, but this extends only to financial liabilities and not to liability for malpractice. Generally speaking, an individual might begin in a sole proprietorship and might at a later date incorporate.

When two or more individuals organize a business, the choices are greater. Some of the same thinking that the single individual follows is applicable here as well. Once aware of the general requirements for all forms of business entities, one is confronted with choosing the best one for one's own situation. If there is one person, there are only two choices: a sole proprietorship or a corporation.

Now you find a place to open up your office, and there are a lot of headaches in that. You have to have a checking account. You need furniture and equipment. You need stationery. You need letterheads. You need business cards and a telephone. Integrated with all of this there must be some kind of accounting system.

Accounting

It is important at the beginning of your career in the business world to hire some kind of professional. It is important to get a lawyer, too, if you have a business form other than a sole proprietorship. If you are in a partnership, you should have a written partnership agreement. This ensures that what you both wanted to get out of the partnership originally, when things were bad, is the same thing you will get a year later when things are better. You will say then, "I thought I was going to get a lot more." It happens all the time in businesses. People forget when they are rich how little they originally wanted; when they are rich they see only how much more they want. A lawyer should write down at the early stages what you both agree on; you sign it, and that document stands until you decide that another one is necessary. It is important that a lawyer help you define your scope based on what has occurred. Whatever the additional cost in having a CPA, it is worth it in getting organized. The biggest problem with small businesses is that when they open they are undercapitalized.

Your accountant will set up that very first budget and advise you on how to record all your expenses and all your income, so that at the end of the year you can bring it to the accountant to have your tax return prepared, provided you do not do it yourself.

If you are a sole proprietor you have the responsibility of reporting all this income, all the receipts and expenses, on Schedule C of the 1040 tax form. Schedule C is for income from professional business. In addition to that you will have to file, assuming you make a net profit, a Schedule SE, which is for self-employment tax. When you are on your own, you have no employer taking out FICA taxes; you as an individual are responsible for paying them. In 1975, if you worked for an employer, he took out 5.8 percent of your salary up to $14,300; if you were self-employed, you had to pay 6.9 percent. When you are an employee, the employer matches your 5.85 percent, making a total of 11.7 percent; but as an individual you have to file that on a Schedule SE. You can get this form from any Internal Revenue Service office.

If you are in a partnership, the partnership has to file a special tax return, a partnership return, form 1065. Included in this form are the partners' individual forms, called K-1. As indicated earlier, all partnerships are not equal. You may have a 60:40 relationship, or a 90:10 relationship. Or if you have a limited partnership, which means that some partners are not active in the business and have only an investment in the business, such partners get a return on their investment only after certain goals are met, as spelled out by the partnership agreement that was signed at the conception of the organization. The K-1 form will say that if there was $10,000 profit and you had 70 percent of the partnership, then $7000 would be taxable to you and $3000 to the other partner. This is filed annually and requires no tax payment. It's just an information return.

If you have a corporation, the corporation must file a tax return. If it is a corporation for profit it must file a form 1120. It may or may not have a tax liability, depending on the creativity of the accountant involved. Generally speaking, on these closely held, mama-and-papa-type corporations, at year's end in November you figure the profit and loss and determine if there is a profit. It is often recommended by the board of directors, which is made up of you, that at the end of the year a bonus be given or a charitable contribution made, coincidentally equal to the anticipated profit, so you have a very minor taxable income. The reason for this is to avoid double taxation. If the corporation is taxed and a recipient employee of the corporation who is also its owner is taxed, there is double taxation. If you let the corporation pay taxes and give a dividend or profit into a larger salary next year, the recipient will have to pay taxes a second time on basically the same money. If you can adjust salaries and/or bonuses by the end of the year, and they both break even, creating a small loss or a small taxable profit, the accountant is probably doing a good job for you.

Another kind of corporation is the nonprofit corporation. This entails more legal expenses and more legal filing. The corporation does not pay an income tax, but there are a lot more regulations involved. The rules are basically the same as for profit-making corporations.

A third type of corporation is a subchapter S corporation. This means that you have a corporate entity. You have all the liability protection of a corporation, but the tax liability is based on flow-through theory. All the taxable income goes through the corporation to the 1120S corporation (subchapter S corporation) and is taxed to the individual stockholders based on the percentages of outstanding stock they own (similar to a partnership). A subchapter S corporation is often best for the first couple of years in business because of some very specific tax benefits such as investment credit. The flow-through theory allows you to get all the tax benefits in the early stages of the corporation. There is usually no money made in the first couple of years; so you get a loss on your principal tax return benefits of investment credit using certain tax loopholes. They are allowed by the Internal Revenue Service. Then when it starts to make money, you elect to go to a regular corporation, but in the meantime you have had the best of both worlds.

Sources of Helpful Information

There are sources of information that can help you in starting your business other than a professional person. The Small Business Administration (SBA) is a government agency that provides free service to anybody who wants to open any kind of business. People with whom you can set up an appointment to advise you on your business will set up a budget for you. They will meet with you after a month, 2 months, 3 months, and a year, and they will assist you in your business and give you good business advice. The SBA also publishes about 50 pamphlets, available without charge, that are good sources of documented information. Titles of some of the most useful ones are as follows:

1. Legal and Accounting Services for a Service Firm
2. Record Keeping Systems
3. Choosing the Legal Structure of Your Firm
4. Checklist for Going into Business
5. Budgetary Requirements
6. Employee Benefit Plans
7. Cash Management and Borrowing

Opening an Office

Once you have decided to go into the private sector and have defined the service you have to offer, developed the capital needed, secured the necessary legal and economic counsel, and determined the business structure that is best for you, you will need to open an office. Some of the other areas that I believe nurses opening an office for themselves need to consider are these:

1. A place to do business
2. Furniture and equipment
3. Letterheads and business cards
4. Insurance
5. Hiring and firing
6. Billing and accounts receivable
7. Paying bills
8. A business checking account with working capital

Finding an adequate place to locate your business involves looking for a centrally located neighborhood and an office building with an elevator, if you are on other than the main floor. You will have older people, people in wheelchairs, and people who are young but who have respiratory problems and can't walk up even one flight of stairs. You will need a lease, which your attorney should review. Check for adequate lavatory facilities and adequate parking. Plan on paying the first month's rent and last month's rent plus a security deposit.

Once a location has been found, it must be furnished with desks, sofas, chairs, lamps, typewriter, filing cabinets, and other equipment, all of which require money. Go out to the discount houses and determine how much each will cost. You are going to need them. You need stationery and letterhead and business cards. Determine your legal name. Go to a stationery house and find out how long it takes to get stationery. Give them all the information and tell them when you would like the order. Call the telephone company and find out when they are putting out the new Yellow Pages. Tie up your telephone immediately, even though you may not need it for 6 months, so that you will be in the Yellow Pages. The telephone company often wants a security deposit; if you are responsible for utilities, utility companies may want security deposits. By the time you are ready to conduct business you should have contacted an insurance agent to review all insurance needs: malpractice, liability, lease, automobile, and industrial.

The size of your firm will dictate whether you need any other employees. When you first start you may not need an employee, and in a partnership you may never need one. Usually the first employee needed is a secretarial assistant to answer the telephone and do the typing. The interviewing process is a very important area that often is discounted by new employers. You ought to sit down before you interview anybody and write out the scope of the job and the responsibilities. Write as if you were going in for the job: What do you want to know? What are the fringe benefits? What are the hours? What is the salary? What are the working conditions? What are the sick-pay conditions? What about promotion? Have it all written, because firing is a by-product of poor interviewing, generally speaking. It's very difficult to fire someone, even when the person deserves to be fired. Interviewing is especially important in a small office, because your one or two employees will be seen as an extension of you, and your clients will give you some of the credit for what they do, as well as all the blame.

Regardless of what you call your business entity, you must be able to account for all monies coming in and going out, which means you need a bookkeeping system. In order to report this information to the different government agencies you will need government identification numbers. You may need state and federal identification numbers and, depending on your state, other numbers related to your payroll reporting requirements. Some cities require you to have a business license, and some professional state agencies also require you to obtain a license.

In setting up the financial aspects of business operation, my responsibilities as an accountant are quite specific. We have rules in the accounting profession. Although nurses may come to my group and say, "We need your help," they are still just another business to me. We have certain ground rules that all business organizations have to follow. They have to have an accounting system. They have to have an organization. They have to keep track of their money. They have to keep track of what is owed to them and what money is spent, which means they have to have a bookkeeping system. There are some very finite rules, and this certainly makes it easier for me.

In the beginning, bookkeeping can be simplified; so you can do it. At the end of the year the CPA goes through it and puts together the financial statement as well as the tax returns. Then it is filed. It is only on special occasions that you have to go to the CPA, eg, if you need a bank loan, if you want to review your budget, if you want an adjusted trial balance or a profit-and-loss statement to see where you are and where you are going. Most organizations have the right to use either the accrual or the cash basis in keeping accounts. This is a decision you have to make. Most professional people do not deal on the accrual basis. You perform a service today and you bill it out, but you may not get paid for 30 days. If you were on the accrual basis, you would record that money as if you had already received it. You would record it as income as soon as the statement went out, and you would pay taxes on it even though you had not received it; the same would be true for accounts payable. In this system you record your commitments. You buy some office supplies in December, but you will not get a bill until January and will not pay it until February; nevertheless, you record it in the month you transact the business. The disadvantage of this system for the professions is that you have a high rate of uncollectables as well as slow payment on accounts receivable. If you used the accrual basis you would be paying taxes on monies you had not received or would not receive. Most people use the cash basis. You may have a supplementary accounting system to keep track of the money owed to you; if you do not get that money, you may as well close up shop. The bookkeeping system also will provide for billing clients as well as paying bills.

To perform all the foregoing tasks, you must have a checking account with adequate working capital integrated with a cash-required projection and a flexible budget. Do not write checks out of your personal account. It is very difficult to control your bookkeeping system if you are paying your house bills, food bills, and office bills out of the same account. All these things cost money, and you might not have any income for 3 or 6 months. The expenses start yesterday. If you decide to open a business yourself, as opposed to going to somebody to help you, you ought to sit down and plan a budget. The average salaried employee, whether professional or not, is usually not aware of the problems and paperwork involved with opening up a business.

But even with all that is required, I thoroughly believe that the rewards, both financial and personal, far outweigh the additional responsibilities and paperwork. I believe that if you sit down and carefully map the necessary steps for moving into the private sector of business, plan your time and your moves, you will be rewarded for your efforts.

DISCUSSION

MAXINE BARDACH: My interest is learning more about insurance.

LARRY SUBRIN: Before you open your office you have to establish a relationship with an insurance man. You have to find a full-service insurance agent. You want to be sure they know their business, because you are involved with liability, malpractice, and industrial insurance. Those are very specialized areas. Your life insurance agent is usually just a salesman, and you need somebody who is going to give you service. An accountant knows that you need certain insurances and can tell you if the fees involved are representative of what other clients are paying. Industrial insurance covers injuries on the job. If a sole practitioner is hurt on the job, nobody helps you. If a partner in a general partnership is hurt on the job, nobody helps. But if an employee of a corporation is hurt, insurance through this industrial insurance covers you. There is some income protection; the corporation has paid for it at a very reasonable premium that an individual cannot get. An individual can get a kind of insurance called income continuation. For example, you have $1500 or $2000 worth of income protection, which means that if you are hurt and away from the job for a week then the insurance company will pay you, but you pay a very steep premium for that insurance. It is really insurance for your family. Industrial insurance costs substantially less. Also, the entire amount of industrial insurance is tax-deductible, while income continuation insurance is not deductible in any way. But neither the insurance premium nor the income is taxable in either case. It is important to find out about insurance before opening your office, because it very often is a big expense, and depending on the agent and your relationship with him, all the premium may have to be paid in advance, which could be substantial. Doctors pay anywhere from $1000 to $2000 per month, and the insurance companies want 6 months advance. If that happens to nurses (and nurses are having some trouble getting malpractice insurance) they are going to have the same prepayment problems. It is very important to look into insurance coverage. Your accountant can advise you on cost factors.

Sometimes when you are starting out and cannot afford income continuation insurance, you can get insurance to protect your ongoing expenses. Overhead insurance guarantees that your income will not have to be used to offset the costs of continuation of business. You can get that in a partnership or as an individual. . . .

EVELYN CHAPMAN: If you have somebody working by the hour, maybe a couple of hours a week to help fill in, what do you have to cover them under?

LARRY SUBRIN: In Arizona I recommend to my clients that they pay as any employee and cover for Social Security. This means you should take out all withholding taxes, federal, state, and city, if there are any. In Arizona one or more employees have to be covered. That changed in 1974; it used to be three or more. It is also true in Arizona that if you are a corporation and you fire yourself you can get unemployment insurance, which you can't get if you fire yourself in a partnership or in a sole proprietorship. In Arizona you have to pay for that if you have one or more employees. When you hire an employee you should add approximately 10 percent to the cost of his salary for other expenses associated with his employment. If you hire a person for $1000 per month, it costs you a lot of money, because you have Social Security, industrial insurance, and sometimes a little health and accident insurance. The benefits are approximately 10 percent. A nonprofit corporation is automatically exempt from the Social Security requirement. If they want to elect to go into it they can. If they elect to go in, it means they are committed for 10 years. The advantage is that you do not have any Social Security withholding, and you just saved yourself approximately 6 percent on salaries. . . .

PARTICIPANT: Pursuant to that, would you comment on the sole proprietor Social Security requirements?

LARRY SUBRIN: In 1975 Congress passed the Individual Retirement Act, which says that if you are self-employed or work for an entity that does not provide a profit sharing or pension plan, you can contribute up to 15 percent of your salary or earnings up to $1500 into a plan and get a deduction for it on your individual income tax return. Insurance companies sell these plans. Stock brokerage houses sell them. Savings and loan associations sell them. If you're not concerned about growth, go into a savings and loan. If you have many working years ahead of you, then go into an insurance company plan, because their rates of return are high. They can give you more because they are not governed by the state banking laws. If you are under 40 years of age, go the insurance route; above age 40, in general, you ought to go the savings and loan route. They will guarantee 6 or 7 percent on your money, and you can figure what it will be in 20 years. I recommend it to all my clients. It's a tax gift, and it's usually within reach of most of us. I went in and borrowed the $1500 to pay for the plan. I paid the $1500 back at $150 per month over the next year, and I get a tax deduction of the interest; so I've leveraged it and have not used any of my money. You can do the same thing. Some savings and loan associations will set up a loan to let you buy a plan; so you do not necessarily have to come up with your own money.

I have a client who went to the bank the other day and borrowed $10,000 to make his commitment to a nonprofit organization. Specifically, he made a commitment of $15,000. He had already paid $5000 and he went to the bank to borrow the $10,000 so that he could get a deduction in 1975 for $15,000. $5000 of it came out of his current income. He was in the 60 percent bracket, so that means that $10,000 only cost him $4000. He saved $6000 through Uncle Sam. Those are the kind of tax planning things that are done at the end of the year between October and December with your accountant if you are in the 40 percent range and above. Do not ever go into a tax shelter if you're not in the 50 percent range. . . .

PARTICIPANT: I have two questions. Is there any advantage if you are already in a Keough plan to change it to something else?

LARRY SUBRIN: The Keough plan in the past has been heavily into the stock market, but if you have made contributions greater than $1500 and you're in a more evenly invested type (if the investment is not primarily in the stock market), I'd say don't get out of the Keough plan, because that gives you higher limitation. . . .

PARTICIPANT: OK. The other question is this: If I have a salary with a fringe benefit, how can I estimate how much more I need to make without a salary to cover that fringe benefit?

LARRY SUBRIN: Well, I'll tell you what the rule of thumb is in the accounting office. When you hire somebody, you should charge to that person about three times what you pay him. If you hire somebody and pay him $100 per week, or about $2.50 per hour for a 40-hour week, you add 10 percent to that, because that's the fringe benefits; so it's $2.75 per hour. You want to see that he is productive to the extent that he is earning you about three times what you are paying him.

PARTICIPANT: That's not what I asked you.

LARRY SUBRIN: I didn't understand your question.

PARTICIPANT: How much do I need to net to compensate for providing my own fringe benefits?

LARRY SUBRIN: Let me see if I understand.

PARTICIPANT: If I have a salary of $16,000 plus fringe benefits, how much more do I need to make on my own, what percentage?

LARRY SUBRIN: OK, I understand the question. There is no specific answer for that because there are too many unknown factors. That is one of the things a CPA would sit down and work out with you. He will tell you that if you want to make $16,000 when you are through, that is really $18,000 with fringe benefits. That is based on the numbers (how much your rent is, how much your costs are) that we know about. I would have to know the other numbers and figure it to be accurate. It is not any given percentage, because there are so many other factors.

PARTICIPANT: But you quickly added $2000 to that $16,000.

LARRY SUBRIN: Well, I said you considered your fringe benefits as $2000. I just arbitrarily did that. There's really no specific number in there. I'd love to answer your question, and I'm not trying to beat around the bush, but every one of you can have a different figure. . . .

PARTICIPANT: Do you do the same service and charge one person one price and another person another price?

LARRY SUBRIN: It isn't the same service. I really do not find any problem with that as long as I do not charge a great deal more because someone is wealthy. In other words, I have a fee range; I do free things, and I do things at the bottom of the range. No client can tell me he has or does not have money; I'm in a position to know. He is not fooling anybody. If a client lies to me the lie is obvious as soon as I get the books. Then I would just as soon he go somewhere else, because it is not going to work. You have to have good rapport with your CPA and your lawyer. Those two people, for a developing firm, can contribute more than anyone else. I try to move beyond clients who want to use me for the bookkeeping function. I would like clients to use me as a true professional. In Nursing Care and Consultation we got involved in negotiating a contract with the government not too long ago. We studied their requirements, and then we set up our books and our proposal to comply almost to the letter with their requirements. In fact, because we were so efficient I think they even changed their requirements to a certain degree to comply with us. They use me for that, and they use their lawyer to review very technical documents, but they are very adept. Janet (Nusbaum) and Nancy (Keller) do all the homework. I always thought anybody in the medical field was very poor at business. Doctors and dentists are usually terrible. They know how to charge, but they do not know what to do with the money when they get it. I found from my limited experience with nurses in Tucson that they are very astute and their questions are very intelligent. Sometimes they make me squirm a little because I don't have the answer. That's the way it ought to be. You should get your money's worth. Thirty-five dollars per hour should not be thrown away, and that is what they pay. If you are not happy with the service or don't have trust in your CPA, there is no reason to keep on. The door swings both ways. . . .

PARTICIPANT: Do you have any suggestions for women going into business? How do you select a CPA? What sorts of things do you look for in selecting an accountant?

LARRY SUBRIN: I would interview him just as I would interview anybody else. I'd tie down the question of fees and ask, "Do you charge for telephone calls? Do you charge for lunches?" Make sure that when your accountants send you a bill they do not say "monthly billing." Tell them you want an itemized bill. Find out what they can do for you and what they expect from you. Generally speaking, when I have new clients come in I tell them about my background. I am always very careful to tell them what my background is so that they can see that I am not all serious. I'm serious about my work, but I do not come across that way, and I tell them about my family because I think that's important. I tell them I am going to stay there. I tell them about my philosophy. I don't cheat and I don't expect them to, and if they do they don't get me involved; as soon as I'm involved I give up their account. I don't need it, and I tell them that. I mean, that's nobody's business, and certainly don't tell a secretary. I sit down and I tell them that if I don't get what I expect they're just going to pay for the difference. They ought to have enough appreciation for the money they spend to follow the advice, and if they don't agree with the advice then they ought to go elsewhere. It is just that simple. I have a service I sell. In Tucson we are fortunate because most of the CPA's are very good; if I lose somebody I am not unhappy about it because I'm pretty sure that he will be lucky enough to get somebody good. But that is not true in all cities. You can ask a CPA to give you the names of some of his clients. Call them. Tell them that you talked to the CPA who does their work, and ask if they are satisfied. Often women are taken advantage of, and if they want to get a loan at the bank they better get somebody to help them, because they are going to have more difficulty. They will have more difficulty than a man with the same balance sheet. There is no question about it.

SHARON GEDAN: Some of us have some feelings about women challenging this kind of institution. When I went for a loan I insisted that I get it on my own name, but I had a lawyer prepared to back me up in case of difficulty.

PARTICIPANT: With the new credit law that came into effect October 1, 1975, no woman should ever have any problem getting credit.

PARTICIPANT: I have four or five employees, all of whom are women, because women do much better work at that level. I haven't found anybody to get together with for the betterment of my organization; so I don't have a partner. But should I incorporate?

LARRY SUBRIN: A corporation is really one of the options. It used to be that one could incorporate as soon as he started grossing the big dollars to have the benefits of a pension plan and a profit sharing plan and all the other benefits that one has in a corporation. But you have the money to incorporate (about $1500). Today, with the vagueness of the new pension laws and the new profit sharing laws as well as the lack of a new IRS definition, that advantage has gone out the window. Very few corporations are going into profit sharing plans, because the government will not say what is allowable. This means that 5 years from now they might allow the deduction and they might not. Now it is less desirable to go into a corporation for that specific reason. In addition to the cost of incorporating, you are more restricted. You have to do more things. You have to have more means. You have to document more things. On the other hand, a corporate entity is a lot easier to perpetuate. As you get older and you want to involve new people, it is easier to sell a piece of paper that says you have a share of this corporation. It is more tangible with a corporation. It is an identifiable unit. A corporation has a lot of selling points. While it limits financial liability, that is not so important to professionals. It will not protect you from malpractice. You are open to malpractice whether you are in the corporation or not. . . .

PARTICIPANT: In my case I have a colleague at work. He shares the office, and we split office expenses, but we have no formal partnership. We have our own individual billing and accounts. What would be the advantages of having a partnership?

LARRY SUBRIN: All you have is an association. You just own an office together. I'm not too sure in your case that there would be any advantage in a partnership. Do your consumers think that you're a partnership?

PARTICIPANT: No, they usually come to us because of our individual reputations. Once in a while we refer to each other.

LARRY SUBRIN: You may have reached all the mutual benefits that you will ever want this way. A lawyer might tell you that if it appears that you have a partnership, your patients on a malpractice suit may have the right to sue you because of the appearance of a partnership. Since it crossed my mind as a layman, it might cross theirs. Their lawyer may suggest suing you both, honestly believing that you are a partnership. That may create a legal problem for you. You may want to talk to your own lawyer about it. What does your letterhead say?

PARTICIPANT: We have our own letterheads.

LARRY SUBRIN: In no way do you have both your names in one place? When clients come into your office, are both names on the window?

PARTICIPANT: Yes.

LARRY SUBRIN: That is misleading enough, it seems to me.

PARTICIPANT: We will live with that because we like to work together. . . .

PARTICIPANT: We went the corporation route because we are a vocation business and we're dealing with the University of California, a variety of junior colleges, and health agencies. Government agencies definitely want a corporation, and preferably a nonprofit one. In the by-laws of some of the organizations with which we deal it states that they can contract only with certain kinds of orgnizations. So when we were starting to talk about this initially, our attorney recommended a corporation.

LARRY SUBRIN: You are a 501C corporation?

PARTICIPANT: Right.

LARRY SUBRIN: Have you elected to take out Social Security?

PARTICIPANT: No, we are using IRA. We are not taking out Social Security. In California, if you are willing to do the homework, you can incorporate for less than the average state.

LARRY SUBRIN: I do not think you ought to. I have just seen too many mistakes. That first document is so important, and I'm not trying to make business for the lawyer. That first document could create havoc later on if you have done it wrong. It could create all kinds of problems. Also, if you incorporate and are nonprofit, the goodwill that you build up all the years that you work is not salable. You cannot sell anything; so all the effort you put in will have no dividend 20 years from now. I would not recommend a nonprofit corporation, generally speaking, for the reason that you are putting your whole life into it. When it is all over with you ought to get something out of it—like me when I can sell my practice.

REIMBURSEMENT FOR SERVICES

There is no area that causes greater conflict for nurses moving into the public sector than that of money. While they recognize that this is a capitalistic society, that hospitals are the third largest business in the United States, and that most physicians are extremely successful entrepreneurs (in 1974 the average income of self-employed physicians was $45,146 after subtracting tax-deductible professional expenses),[1] many nurses are still emotionally paralyzed when it comes to considering nursing in any kind of monetary terms. This paralysis is supported at the federal level, by concern for the millions of people who cannot afford health care and the inequitable distribution of health care workers.

Other aspects of the long conflict concern the value of services given by women, the long-existing low self-image that pervades the nursing discipline, the attitudes and pressures exerted by physicians and hospital administrators to play down the value of nursing services, and the public's concern with rising costs.

Within the profession, the fee-for-service concept is considered outmoded when applied to nursing services, despite the fact that most other health professionals earn all or part of their income in this way. Reimbursement for services has become the respectable term, and it apparently links money and service in ways that the fee-for-service concept does not.

Federal legislation will be related to reimbursing health professionals for delivering health care to those deprived of it. If the fee-for-service concept remains the model of payment for medical care, and some other kind of reimbursement for service obtains for nursing care, it is possible that there could become two systems of health care.

Self-serving is the term applied to nurses who are interested in fee for service and third-party payments. One nurse speaks on the point:

It is very possible that nurse practitioners will lean toward health care delivery models that are based on fee for service. They will then end up under the pressures of the reality, doing the same things that are being criticized on the legislative scene. At a time when we are trying to do away with fee for service and its consequences (the maldistribution of health services) it seems that fee for service moves nursing toward aggravating the problems of health care delivery. It promotes the private incentive, which means nurses will go where people can afford to pay.

She continues:

Both physicians and nurses should be on a salary basis. If the nurses are on salary and the physicians on fee for service, the physicians play the old profit game. In joint practice you have the same problem.

Another nurse speaks on the issue this way:

Eight hundred thousand nurses are not going to work individually or independently with Congress saying who is a qualified person for individual reimbursement. We can really abandon this fee-for-service semantics and just talk about reimbursement, which is more meaningful and gets us off the defensive. As a group we should agree to that. The issue is this: Are we as a group of professionals going to stick together sufficiently to arrive at criteria that we can all agree with and submit, ourselves, to attain this reimbursement?

"Increasing the scope of reimbursable services" is the respectable, altruistic way to get paid for nursing care through third-party payers. Again, other arguments for getting paid for one's work are called self-serving. Our conflicts about money persist, while we see other health professionals push legislation increasing fees and other benefits related to Medicare and Medicaid, one after the other. Nurses are beginning to take a position related to getting their fair share of the health care dollar, as other professionals have for years, whether or not they get fee for service. Some members of the group play the devil's advocate in opening up the area of payment for services for nurses in private practice, nurses in joint practice with physicians, and some nurses in independent practice. Putting a monetary value on one's nursing care is an unfamiliar and often very uncomfortable activity for nurses, as already noted. It is considerably more complex than it appears from a distance. One nurse reports:

Part of my problem is identifying what out of all the things I do is work. We are nurses and we have given a lot, but what is the monetary value of what we do? I wish I had a penny for every phone consultation I do. It always starts out with, "I want you to tell me what to do." And then they tell me their problem. Many times it is self-care, but they want to be told to do it or supported to try it. Sometimes I have to see them or advise them to see their physician. Sometimes I just reassure them that they can wait until the morning, when they can come to the office. This takes up a lot of my time, but I do not charge for it.

Another nurse says:

I remember when I was first out of school. You wouldn't think of being paid for taking somebody's blood pressure anywhere. Any nurse who did this might be cited by the nurses' association. During the past 12 years in my state nurses have learned that the legal powers that be cannot threaten anyone for getting paid for providing a service. This is still a revelation to some nurses. If anyone contests your right to be paid for your services, you have the option and the right to return legal action to protect yourself.

There are others who are disconcerted to see nurses paid by the visit or by service unit. One nurse who works in a physician's office in one state has a part-time practice in her hometown several miles away:

In the office setting I'm salaried, but at home I get fees for my services. There are some rumblings by physicians in the area, and some are upset that the money does not go back to the physician and come back to me through him as salary.

Fee Schedules and Salaries

Fees nurses charge vary greatly. Services they offer vary greatly, too. Many nurses charge at the same rate as physicians in the area, on the basis that they perform their functions as well as physicians perform theirs. In general, family nurse practitioners in private practice charge $7 to $15 per visit, plus mileage, especially if travel distance is a matter of miles. They charge, in addition, for the cost of treatments. Home visits are usually $10 or $15 for the first hour, and weekend or night visits may be as high as $15 or $20. Some rates are higher, especially if background data must be collected from other professionals or if considerable communication must be undertaken on the client's behalf. Generally, fees in urban areas are higher than in rural areas, and the first visit may be charged at a higher rate than subsequent visits. Psychiatric nurse practitioners' fees are usually higher, ranging from $15 to $35 per hour for individual care and less for group therapy. Psychiatric nurses also may charge more for the first or intake visit and for evening and night visits. Some psychiatric nurse practitioners do not make home visits, while others think of home visits as one of the unique and most valuable aspects of practice. The greater cost of home visits in terms of the nurse's time is a great concern to some psychiatric nurses. Occasionally a nurse practitioner will rent equipment at rates that are prorated in terms of cost, depreciation, insurance, repair, etc. Table 1 shows the fee schedules of several nurses in private practice from various parts of the country and several salaries of independent nurse practitioners who are salaried.

Salaries for those nurses in joint practice with physicians and those practitioners salaried by the employing agency vary widely, eg, $12,000 to $40,000 per annum. If there are physician's assistants in the area, the nurses strive to at least match their salaries. In rural areas where there are no physician's assistants, salaries seem to be lower. No salary figures are available for practitioners employed in large clinics or medical centers.

Third-Party Payers

As difficult as putting a monetary value on one's services may be, getting approval for payment of nursing services under clients' health care insurance or other coverage is even more difficult from several points of view. One nurse reports: "I don't get involved in third-party pay because I am not going to deal with the paperwork." Others have the same feelings and do the same thing:

> Nurses want to practice. They have little interest or patience with paperwork. They also have little stamina for or persistence in working with insurance commissioners, insurance companies, social welfare departments, and the like to increase the scope of reimbursable costs.

The most difficult payers for nurse practitioners are Blue Cross/Blue Shield and Medicare. Both plans require a physician's signature before they will pay for care. Nurses in solo practice without office assistance complain that the Medicare correspon-

Table 1. Fee Schedules

STATE	TYPE OF PRACTICE	INITIAL OFFICE VISIT	REGULAR OFFICE VISIT	HOUSE CALL	EVENING VISIT	WEEKEND VISIT	MILEAGE
Arizona	General	$10–$25	$5 minimum	$15–$30	No data	No data	No data
Illinois	Psychiatric	$25/individual	$25/individual	No data	No data	No data	No data
Illinois	Family	No data	$5	$15	No data	No data	No data
Iowa	Psychiatric –mental health (sex counseling)	$20	$10–20	—	$10–$20/hr	—	No home visits
Maryland	Family nurse, Pediatrics	$6 for 15 min; $10 for 30 min	$6 for 15 min; $10 for 30 min	No home visits	No data	No data	No home visits
Massachusetts	Psychiatric –mental health		$35	$35	No data	No data	Client pays travel time
Minnesota	Psychiatric –mental health	$25	$20	$20	$15 for 30 min	$15 for 30 min	No data
South Dakota	Family	No data	No data	$5 for 30 min (9 A.M.–5 P.M.)	$10	$10	Yes
Tennessee	Family	$7	$7	$10			Over 5 miles
Wyoming	Family	$12.50–$45	$5–$37.50	$18.75–$31.25	Regular fees plus $6.25	Regular fees plus $6.25	No data

dence is hardly comprehensible, with a language all its own, and is very time-consuming. One practitioner handles this by making as a condition of her acceptance of clients that they ascertain that their physicians are willing to work with the nurse. If he is not, she will not accept the patient. When there is the need for the physician's signature to get reimbursed for services given under a client's insurance policy, the client gets the physician's signature. Other nurses in private practice have backup physicians who will sign insurance forms. One hopeful sign for nursing is that very few insurance carriers now require that the person who signs the form be the person who delivered the care. What does happen is that the person signing the form, who guarantees that the care was given and given properly, may not have seen the client or may have seen him only in a cursory way, as one nurse exemplifies:

> Clients in the clinic who are ADC patients who are carried on Title 19 can be intakes to the clinic by anyone (a social worker, nurse psychotherapist), but within a certain period of time they have to be seen by an M.D., a psychiatrist. If they are not evaluated by a psychiatrist, then Title 19 will not pay for them. You can imagine how it's handled. Just to fit the criteria of Title 19 carriers, the psychiatrist says, "Hi, how are you today? Good-bye." Seeing a psychiatrist is an unnecessary and costly step in many cases. The taxpayer is charged $25 unnecessarily for a psychiatric evaluation when there is no need for it.

As costs of care are trimmed and wasteful practices are eliminated, this may be one area nurse practitioners can open up for the profession.

Extending the Scope of Reimbursable Services

Nurse practitioners in many areas have focused on trying to keep clients in their case load from the point of view of economics. Convinced of the value of their nursing services, they have moved politically to assure payment for these services by third-party payers, thereby relieving clients of the burden of paying not only for health care insurance but also paying out of pocket for health care. Nurses have worked as individuals, as participants within corporate entities, as members of councils of advanced practitioners, as members of state nurses associations, and as members of various committees, councils, and commissions within the American Nurses Association to get reimbursement for services. They have worked through state insurance commissioners, state departments of welfare, state departments of social services, county boards of health, county welfare departments, and insurance carriers. Some nurses have had considerable success in being paid by insurance companies,* state departments of welfare and social services for Medicaid clients, Title 19 funds, Workman's Compensation, and county welfare departments. Some nurses have obtained contracts with county departments of social services and welfare departments for nursing services.

It is still a problem for nurses to accept the responsibility for being assertive and politically active, but they have no choice if they believe in the value of what they have to offer and if they are not going to penalize the client economically. Getting business licenses and vendor licenses, writing contracts, making grant applications, and securing the various kinds of approvals required to stay in business require tedious, often frustrating work. But these are the facts of going into private practice. The paperwork involved in payment by a third-party carrier is another time-consuming problem. Nurses do not want to nurse papers, but they must find ways, since it is naive at this point in our health care history to think that paperwork will decrease. It is naive to think that nurses are not going to have to learn these aspects of business and join the mainstream of the health care delivery system. It may seem virtuous to reject the nursing of paper, but is it still virtue when the client pays twice for his care?

Contributions to Nurse Practitioners in Private Practice

Despite the concern with fee for service as the way to pay for nursing care, it is important that benefits to the profession not be overlooked. Nurse practitioners in private practice are the nurses who are really setting precedents for nursing in the delivery of health care. First, they are proving that nursing has considerable monetary value. Second, they are meeting a community need that people are willing to pay for personally, even if their insurance will not cover it. Third, they are making some of their contribution with the middle class, which has greater political sophistication and

**Insurance agencies identified by participants as paying them for nursing services: (1) Champus–Military Dependents Insurance (for nurses prepared at the master's level); (2) Workman's Compensation; (3) Medicaid (Public Aid Department, Departments of Welfare and Social Services); (4) Continental National (suture removal); (5) Teachers Retirement (home visits, injections); (6) R.O.M. (counseling, bathing); (7) New York Life (reimbursing client) (bedfast care); (8) American (paraplegic patient); (9) Home Insurance Company (aftercare, psychiatric); (10) Mutual of New York (MONY) (terminal cancer care); (11) State Bank Trust Fund (post polio).*

makes itself heard in legislative circles. Fourth, they are shaking the health care delivery establishment, and they have the potential to completely overhaul it by insisting that the client and the community be listened to, by insisting that health is the basic state to be assessed and supported, and by challenging the traditional pathology-oriented system of medical care as the basic model for health care delivery. Not the least of the challenge is identification of the locus of effective health care delivery. Daily these nurses are extending the scope of reimbursable health care services. Continuation of this kind of activity will ultimately define nursing and provide at least one measure for looking at nursing care.

ECONOMIC AND BUSINESS ASPECTS OF JOINT PHYSICIAN–NURSE PRACTITIONER PRIVATE PRACTICE

Kathleen C. Brown

Nurses prepared to function in expanded roles are increasingly available, and both the health team and the consumer are beginning to recognize and support the utilization of the nurse practitioner to provide primary care services. Nurse practitioners are now employed in outpatient departments, home health or visiting nurse services, health maintenance organizations, and private practice settings. There nurses are expending much time and energy in defining their roles and demonstrating the feasibility of the nurse practitioner as a primary care provider.

To date, two important barriers to implementation of the nurse practitioner role have been identified. Legal barriers have received much attention as state nursing practice acts are studied and revised. Joint practice committees of state nursing associations and state medical societies are discussing the functions appropriate to each discipline and functions that may be shared. The second barrier, the economic aspect, is a comparatively neglected topic. It requires considerable analysis.

In private practice, implementation of the nurse practitioner role is very difficult without adequate planning for the economic and business aspects. Planning for the economics of nurse practitioner services is of increasing concern as administrators, health planners, and nurse practitioners themselves recognize that the viability of this role in private practice settings is dependent on economic factors.

This section will discuss the economic and business aspects of joint physician–nurse practitioner private practice and will propose suggestions for preventing problems that frequently arise in joint practice.

Influence of Economics

The development of a collegial relationship between the two health team members is of utmost importance in a joint physician–nurse practitioner private practice. The nurse expects to participate as a partner with the physician in decision-making and to have the respect of the physician. The physician expects the nurse practitioner to be more vocal and direct in formulating assessments and to assume greater accountability for decisions. These role expectations are essential to joint practice. But one's role is inextricably bound to one's status in the organization. The nurse practitioner who is a salaried employee of a physician will find that the employer–employee relationship promotes a subordinate role for the nurse. Decisions will often be made without the nurse's input. When reminded, the physician will usually indicate that he was unaware that the nurse wanted to be included.

In addition, the degree to which one contributes to attainment of the goals of the organization determines the status, authority, and compensation of that individual.[2] If the primary goal of the practice is to provide acute care services, then the area in which the nurse is particularly adept (ie, health screening, health supervision, education, and care of chronically ill patients) will be designated as having low priority. Less attention will be paid to developing these programs, and the nurse's role will be subordinate to that of the physician when the training and subsequent emphasis are on the care of acutely ill patients. Priority on acute care services is further enhanced by the consumer, who is more inclined to seek acute care services than preventive services. Current reimbursement systems favor payments for acute episodes of illness or injury.

Collegial nurse practitioner–physician relationships in a private practice and the setting of goals consistent with comprehensive health care make avoidance of the employer–employee relationship with a physician advisable. Rather, one of the following arrangements would prove more useful.

The nurse practitioner may become an owner or shareholder in the corporation or may become a partner in a partnership with the physician. In these arrangements the nurse shares the risks as well as the responsibilities of ownership. The nurse will have a financial interest in the organization that is similar to the physician's interest. The nurse will be concerned with the future of the organization and will necessarily be included in decisions. Finally, the nurse will be more assertive and will assume more responsibility for management of the organization. Regulations concerning interdisciplinary professional or medical corporations and partnerships vary from state to state, and legal counsel must be obtained in order to determine how this can best be accomplished. In an established private practice it may be necessary to contract for a junior partnership of 1 or 2 years before buying into the organization. Such an arrangement also gives both parties an opportunity to determine their suitability for joint practice.

In another arrangement the nurse practitioner may contract her services to the physician. The nurse, as an independent, may desire to contract a percentage of all fees generated for nursing services. The percentage is usually 45 to 50 percent for income, and the balance is used for overhead. Until the nurse practitioner has established a clientele and reimbursement mechanisms are developed, the nurse may choose to contract for a guaranteed 6- to 12-month income, then later proceed to the fee-for-service basis.

The foregoing proposed alternatives to the employer–employee relationship of physician and nurse require that the nurse be willing to commit time, energy, and money and that the physician view the joint practice arrangements with favor.

Reimbursement Issues

Some of the many reimbursement questions posed by the joint nurse practitioner–physician private practice are these: Should the nurse practitioner be on a salaried basis or a fee-for-service basis? Should the nurse practitioner be eligible for third-party reimbursement? Should reimbursement be based on the education of the individual? At what percentage of the physician's fees and income should the nurse's fees and income be set?[3] Nurse practitioners who are in joint practice with physicians have to address these issues, often without the assistance of administrators. A third-party administrator can assist nurse and physician in negotiating fair and reasonable fees, income, and reimbursement mechanisms. Since there exists a paradox between the federal government's planning for training of nurse practitioners and its planning for reimbursement of nurse practitioners, considerable study must be undertaken by both nurse and physician to determine the optimum means of reimbursing the nurse. Planning is needed in order to avoid situations in which the nurse practitioner becomes a financial liability. Attention should be given to avoiding underpayment of the nurse in respect to productivity. The nurse who is underpaid may unknowingly be making a profit for the organization.[3]

As to whether the nurse practitioner should be on a salary or on a fee-for-service basis, it is important to refer once again to the desirability of an egalitarian relationship between the nurse practitioner and the physician. If the physician in the private practice is on salary, it may be desirable for the nurse also to be salaried—but only if the nurse has ownership in the corporation or partnership. If the physician's income is based on fee for service and the nurse's income is to be based on nursing fees, then two important obstacles must be surmounted: a market for nursing services must be created, and the difficulties of reimbursement from third-party carriers for nursing services must be overcome.

A market for nurse practitioner services is required in order for the nurse to survive in a fee-for-service system. Most patients and other health care providers have had little or no contact with nurse practitioners, and thus they are unlikely to make direct requests or referrals for nursing services. Unlike the physician, the nurse usually does not build a case load from physician referrals and emergency room pickups. Relying solely on referrals from the physician in the joint practice may result in a limited case load for the nurse. To acquire an adequate case load and to ensure economic viability, it is recommended that as patients telephone for appointments for primary health care services the receptionist make appointments for many of these patients with the nurse practitioner.

The second obstacle is the present limit on reimbursement for nurse practitioner services. Current reimbursement practices allow for reimbursement only when the physician sees the patient during the visit to the nurse practitioner. This system excludes independent visits by nurses in private practice satellites and nursing homes. Nurses who see patients independently in institutional settings that are on a prepaid contract or formula capitation basis do receive reimbursement. Visiting nurses and private duty nurses also receive reimbursement, but these nurses function with physicians' orders. In many instances this exclusion of nurse practitioners is changing, and some nurse practitioners receive reimbursement for their services. Bills are presently in Congress to amend the Social Security Act to provide for inclusion of registered nurse services under Medicare and Medicaid. As already noted, the current system focuses on reimbursement for treatment of episodic illness.[3] The nurse practitioner whose focus is health may find that third-party payers are not reimbursing for health screening, health education, and counseling.

The obstacles that have been described must be recognized by the nurse practitioner as barriers to success in a fee-for-service model. With planning and with time, these obstacles will be minimized.

Another issue is whether reimbursement should be based on the education and training of the individual or on the tasks performed, without respect to educational preparation.[3] Basing reimbursement on the amount of education of the care provider warrants the implication that there are two or more levels of quality of care and that the more it costs the better the quality of the care. Does more education mean better quality? Is it not true that the nurse practitioner monitoring the hypertensive patient must function at and be accountable at the same level as a competent physician?

Those who feel that reimbursement should be based on the reimbursable tasks are neglecting the fact that fee schedules seldom follow rational rules; they derive from tradition, from insurance company rates, and from other imprecise data. Those who say that reimbursement should be based on expertise must remember that the nurse is equally as skilled as the physician in some instances, if not more skilled in some areas. Also, the nurse practitioner, by virtue of comprehensive attention to patients' physical, psychosocial, educational, and counseling needs, usually spends twice as much time with the patient as does the physician. Others feel that fees should be based on the costs of education. Is this valid when the time and expense involved in educating a nurse in this role are increasing, as compared to the trend toward decreasing the years spent by the student in medical education? If reimbursement is to be based on educational costs, then there must be research comparing educational cost to output.[4] To date, the consensus on this issue is that a uniform fee schedule for all health care providers is desirable. This promotes the concept that care of one quality is provided and that the care provided by the nurse practitioner is of the same quality as care provided by the physician.[3]

The next issue is at what percentage of the physician's fees and income the nurse's fees and income should be set. Some arbitrary figures have been proposed, such as that the physician's income should be two to three times the nurse's salary. This fails to take into account that the nurse practitioner is assuming responsibilities that traditionally have been carried by the physician. The nurse managing the hypertensive patient should be justly compensated for assuming this greater responsibility. An example of the fact that increased responsibilities have not resulted in increased compensation is the intensive care nurse who defibrillates and carefully monitors cardiac patients. This nurse has assumed more responsibility but has received no differential; the CCU nurse receives staff nurse wages. In their eagerness to assume expanded roles, nurses are accepting salaries that do not justly reimburse them for their new responsibilities and output. Nursing should oppose the utilization of nurse practitioners in primary care settings as substitutes for physicians. Nurses can very easily be induced to assume similar responsibilities at a fraction of the income that physicians expect. Nursing is predominantly a woman's field with a history of low wages. Nursing can profit from constant reminder of the fact that nurse practitioners are for the most part underpaid. In a study of pediatric nurse associates it was found that these nurses were underpaid in relation to net income generated.[4]

How should income be calculated? Nurse practitioners are as yet unable to produce figures on median incomes of nurse practitioners in their regions; so when the physician proposes that the nurse practitioner's income be based on that of the nurse's peers, the nurse is unable to quote figures (the physician will quickly quote the median income of his peers). Since nurse practitioners are usually underpaid in terms of their responsibilities and output, it is probably not wise to base one's income expectation on the present median income for nurse practitioners.

One way to calculate a reasonable income is by keeping records of patient encounters and doing cost–benefit analyses. For example, determine the gross fees generated from nursing services, and then subtract 40 to 55 percent of total fees for overhead, including administrative costs, clerical and ancillary costs, and initial and continuing costs for consultation with a physician. The resulting figure should be the nurse practitioner's income.

Business Aspects

In a private practice the nurse practitioner is necessarily involved in the business and management aspects of the organization. These business areas include policy-making, personnel supervision, facility maintenance, public relations, finances, planning for future services, and evaluation. Health professionals have been educated to care for patients, but not to care for a business. Developing the skills in management necessary to motivate the staff to be courteous and efficient in making appointments and collecting fees is in itself a difficult task. Also, those responsible for management must decide on the appropriate mix of receptionists, laboratory technicians, and clinical assistants; they must determine salaries for staff and keep the accounts receivable low and collections high; they must maintain the physical facility so that it is clean, well lighted, and at the proper temperature. Add to this complex the challenge of implementing the nurse practitioner role, establishing a nursing case load, developing a collegial relationship with the physician, and getting reimbursed for nursing services and one can appreciate the importance of the nurse practitioner investigating the economic and business aspects of joint practice.

Specific considerations in relation to the business aspects of joint practice need to be identified. First, in the joint practice arrangement it is essential that the nurse assume responsibility for managerial tasks. The tasks should be based on the abilities of the nurse practitioner as well as on the needs of the organization. Nursing input is also valuable in most policy-making in private practice.

There must be a contract that delineates the conditions of joint practice that the nurse practitioner and the physician find acceptable. The contract must specify the following: the nurse's patient care and administrative responsibilities, how fees will be set and reimbursement accomplished, income and benefits, settings in which the nurse will practice, designated ancillary services including clerical and clinical support, how appointments and referrals to the nurse are to be made, physician support and consultation to be expected, and designated joint times for planning. In view of the difficulties in implementing this new role, it is best to be specific at the outset in drawing up the contract.

Finally, the nurse practitioner must be visible in the community. Public relations efforts are necessary to promote the nurse practitioner in private practice, and to accomplish this the nurse's name should appear on the listing of professional practitioners in the lobby and on business cards, stationery, and handouts to patients. Office staff should be able to explain the nurse's role. An explanation sheet for patients may be of benefit in defining the nurse practitioner's role. Announcements to agencies, nurses, physicians, and pharmacists should be sent to publicize the fact that a nurse is involved in the practice. A visit to the local medical facility and involvement in local health care organizations are also very important. The nurse practitioner should seek hospital privileges in order to gain access to patients' charts and should become involved in continuing education activities of the hospital. In the community the nurse should be involved in health planning committees and civic organizations.

Planning for nurse practitioner services requires a thorough understanding of the economic and business aspects of private practice. Economic and business issues and problems and alternatives related to the nurse practitioner role are complex. Through sharing experiences with peers and communicating solutions to problems, the implementation of the nurse practitioner role will be simplified. Joint nurse practitioner–physican private practices can evolve into entities that are enjoyable for patients and beneficial to both groups of professionals.

REFERENCES

1. Farber L: Doctors' earnings: winning the battle, losing the war. Med Econ 52:184, November 10, 1975
2. Zola IK, McKinley JB: Organizational Issues in the Delivery of Health Services. New York, PRODIST, Neale Watson Academic Publications, 1974
3. Cohen ED, Crootof LM, Goldfarb M, Keenan K, Korper MM, Triffin M: An Evaluation of Policy Related Research on New and Expanded Roles of Health Workers. New Haven, Office of Regional Activities and Continuing Education, Yale University School of Medicine, 1974
4. Yankauer A, Tripp S, Andrews P, Connelly JP: The costs of training and the income generation potential of pediatric nurse practitioners. Pediatrics 49:878, 1972

BIBLIOGRAPHY

Brown KC: The nurse practitioner in a private group practice. Nurs Outlook 22:108, February 1974

Lippard VW, Purcell EF (eds): Intermediate-Level Health Practitioners. New York, Josiah Macy, Jr., Foundation, 1973

McKinley JB (ed): Economic Aspects of Health Care. New York, PRODIST, Neale Watson Academic Publications, 1973

Schiff DW, Fraser C, Walters H: The pediatric nurse practitioner in the office of pediatricians in private practice. Pediatrics 44:62, 1969

CHAPTER 7

Perspectives on Professional Practice

Loretta C. Ford

For some weeks I've been considering the conceptual framework of this presentation. The relationships of the various topics seemed at times quite clear and at other times elusive. It was not that any of the aspects were foreign to me; the multifaceted problem of putting together in a tracer method the organizational, legislative, economic, and social aspects of the professional practice of nursing and incorporating the concerns of the women's movement and the professionalization of nursing practice was an interesting exploration of topics I've addressed before. Perhaps familiarity is the problem. Nevertheless, throughout an extensive review of these problems I asked myself, "What can I do to help make this experience meaningful for those I'm committed to serve—you who are the conferees here today?" I decided that I must not help perpetuate the status quo, support professional egos, and make this conference "memorably satisfying" because it validated current platitudes and postures. I hope that what I have to say challenges you to think, to listen openly, to communicate clearly, to argue objectively, to seek out new facts and ideas, and to explore creative ways of addressing larger issues and problems in nursing and health care. It is to be hoped that our individual behaviors will be altered in some way by this conference and that we will address the larger mission of improving health care to our 215 million citizens.

As a beginning, let me present a few opinions:

1. Independent practice, for nurses as well as for all health professionals, is passé, a myth; it is 50 years too late and is not viable in today's evolving health care systems.

2. Nurses are more concerned about reimbursement for their practice than they are about the larger issues in health, ie, national health insurance, interdisciplinary patterns for health care delivery, and the need for research.

3. The majority of nurses have been unwilling to invest what it's going to take to make nursing a significant force in influencing local and national health policy, in enriching nursing education programs, in influencing the quality of nursing and health care delivery, in generating new knowledge through scientific investigation of the effectiveness, efficiency, cost, and humaneness of clinical practice, and in providing better nursing and health care. Note that I'm not talking only about nursing; I'm also talking about health.

4. Registered nurses, even though they are over a million strong in this nation and control more than one-third of the cadre of 4.5 million health workers, lack the broad power base, the experience in leadership, and the knowledge of change processes to influence policy decisions in organizational and legislative matters. Nurses are too clinically oriented, too work-oriented, and too introverted into *nursing* to address the larger problems in the area of national health matters.

So why am I here? In *Fiddler on the Roof* the dairyman Tevye said, in talking very personally to his God, "On the other hand. . . ."

1. Interdependent practice for all health professionals in health care (which has great potential for independent nursing practice and which I really also support) is futuristic, viable, economically feasible, and professionally satisfying.

2. Reimbursement for identifiable nursing services is a necessary component of a well-designed, financially sound health care system.

3. There are nurses in leadership positions in practice, education, and research who have the vision, the dedication, and the intelligence to exert a positive influence on the forces within government, education, and philanthropy that determine national health policy.

4. While nurses themselves do not and need not have a monopoly on expertise, knowledge, and power, there are other people

(notably consumers) who can make considerable contributions. (Don't forget the strength of other women, who are the largest consumers of health care.)

Now, hopefully, I have your attention, which will allow me to address some of the complex issues that have an impact on practice. My strategy in this review is to focus on the present, to dip into the past, and to draw implications for nursing practice for the future. Let's start with legislation.

LEGISLATION

Examining the proposed and the recently enacted federal and state legislation dealing with the training of nurse practitioners and with their nursing practices is a fruitful exercise for anyone pondering the future of nursing. Examples are drawn from three sources: the federal Health Planning and Resources Development Act (PL 93-641), the nurse training and education acts, and those state practice acts that have been altered within the past decade to accommodate new roles for nurses and other types of practitioners in medical and health care. At the federal level the Health Planning and Resources Development Act of 1974 authorized a 3-year program with two new titles under the Public Health Service Act for health planning and resources development (Title XV established the health planning and resources development and Title XVI revised present programs for the construction and renovation of health care facilities and authorized funds for developing health resources). This legislation replaced the Hill-Burton program, the regional medical program, and the comprehensive health planning program; it charges the individual states to designate health service areas, each of which will have a Health Service Agency (HSA).

> The HSA will be generally responsible for preparing and implementing plans designed to improve the health of the residents of its health service area; to increase the accessibility, acceptability, continuity, and quality of health services in the area; to restrain increases in the cost of providing health services; and to prevent unnecessary duplication of health resources.[1]

This new health planning legislation directs the secretary of the Department of Health, Education, and Welfare to "issue guidelines on national health planning policy, provide priorities on health planning goals, and establish a national council on Health Planning and Development."

You may well ask: So what has that to do with our concerns as independent nurse practitioners? Just this: of the priority list of 10 items specified in the law, items 3, 4, 6, 8, and 10 are directly related to nurse practitioner practice and preparation:

1. Primary care services for medically underserved populations, especially in rural or economically depressed areas.
2. Development of multi-institutional systems for coordinating or consolidating institutional health services.
3. Developing medical group practices, health maintenance organizations, and other organized systems for providing health care.
4. Training and increasing utilization of physician assistants, especially nurse clinicians.
5. Developing multi-institutional arrangements for sharing support services.
6. Promoting activities to achieve improved quality in health services.
7. The development by health service institutions of the capacity to provide various levels of care on a geographically integrated basis.
8. Promoting activities for preventing disease, including studies of nutritional and environmental factors affecting health and the provision of preventive health care services.
9. Adopting uniform cost accounting and other improved management procedures for health service institutions.
10. Developing effective methods of educating the general public concerning proper personal health care and effective use of available health services.[1]

The emphasis on planning is a hopeful sign; it is an effort to bring order, direction, and economy to the systems (or nonsystems, if you wish) of health services, education, and research. The public assumes a powerful position in this legislation. Its provisions call for consumer membership of at least one-half on the statewide coordinating councils and local health service agencies. Providers are also eligible for membership, but the intent of the law is clearly to create a balance of power that favors the consumer. When the question, "Who is a consumer?" is asked, the facetious answer has often been, "Anyone who is not a provider of care or a household member of a provider." (That last qualification is an interesting addition when we recall that the health care industry is the second largest business in the country. Its employment ranks are now swelled to almost 5 million. Add the household members of providers who are ineligible and it may take a while to find a bona fide consumer!)

This legislative effort is a prelude to establishment of national health policy that includes regionalization of health service delivery, federal regulation of the education of health workers, and federal influence on health service (and probably clinical) research.

Another matter of considerable importance is the health manpower training legislation that is authorized at federal and local levels. Practitioners should be aware that the new Nurse Training Act provides for both short-term training and advanced-degree education for the preparation of nurse practitioners in continuing education patterns and clinical nurse specialists at the master's degree level. This emphasis requires that nurses carefully review their curriculum plans as they relate to the use of scarce resources, the costs of ambulatory care education, the new interdisciplinary opportunities offered, and the need for faculty retraining and retooling for primary care and other types of care. But this federal legislation at the program level will be for naught if nursing does not maintain its control, monitoring, and evaluation of practice. Further, nursing must find adequate long-range mechanisms for financial reimbursement. Legal control of practice is generally determined in state administrative agencies, usually boards of nursing that administer state statutes. In the past 10 years a number of changes in the statutory law embodied in the nursing practice acts have occurred.[2]

Probably the milestone legislation that was passed in New York on its second introduction in 1972, after a tremendous battle with medical groups, provides the definitive legislative description of the nature of nursing:

> The practice of the profession of nursing as a registered professional nurse is defined as diagnosing and treating human health problems through such services as casefinding, health teaching, health counseling and provision of care supportive to or restorative of life and well-being, and executing medical regimens prescribed by a licensed or otherwise legally authorized physician or dentist. A nursing regimen shall be consistent with and shall not vary any existing medical regimen.[3]

As opposed to the traditional legal definition of nursing, which distinguished between independent (observing, counseling, teaching, and supervision of others) and dependent acts (administering medications and medical therapies), the New York Practice Act definition does make conceptual distinctions. Some people have been critical of the part of the definition that deals with the limitation that the nursing regimen "shall be consistent with and shall not vary any existing medical regimen," arguing that a profession has no dependent functions, especially not functions that are dependent on medicine.

Some nurses in New York believe that the final phrase is anathema to professional nursing practice, and indeed it may be. Having not been part of the team of nurses who actively furthered the legislation, I can only report that the interpretation is that many patient care plans are shared between professionals, and in the long run it should be the patient, not the provider, who makes the choices.

I would argue that all health professions, including nursing, have no choice but to be interdependent if society is to be well served in health care. Professional providers must learn to collaborate and coordinate their efforts if they hope to survive and flourish. I would further argue that in attempting to be successfully independent our main problems in nursing are not related to identification of tasks and functions but in defining *conceptually* (ie, abstractly as opposed to concretely) the nature of nursing. After we make that definition, then the processes, legal and other, that determine the scope of practice can be successfully identified and implemented.

As the scope of practice in nursing has begun to expand, other states have promulgated statutory changes in nursing practice acts to accommodate these new roles. Late in the 1960s Idaho passed an amendment to the nursing and medical practice acts that created a joint practice board. Many other states followed that lead. Hall's work provides an excellent review of these changes during the past decade.[2]

But with all these and other legal changes and the subsequent reinterpretation of the nurse's role, I sometimes feel a bit uneasy. The uneasiness derives from the misinterpretation and lack of understanding of the statutes on the part of some nurses and laymen. Theoretically the intent of the law is, first of all, to protect the public, and changes to increase the scope of practice ought to be begun from an already well-conceptualized model that considers the nature of practice. The interpretation of the scope of practice ought to address the issues of roles, relationships, and responsibilities, not tasks and functions.

The nature of nursing is beautifully described by Henderson.[4] She postulates a philosophic commitment to caring for and about people of all ages and formulates a conceptual base for practice:

> The unique function of the nurse is to assist the individual, sick or well, in the performance of those activities contributing to health or its recovery or to a peaceful death that he would perform unaided if he had the necessary strength, the will or independence as rapidly as possible. . . . This concept of the nurse as a substitute for what the patient lacks (not what the physician lacks) to make him "complete," "whole," or "independent" . . . may seem limited to some. The more one thinks about it, however, the more complex the nurse's function as so defined proves to be. Think how rare is "completeness," or "wholeness," of mind and body, to what extent it is acquired, but it is generally admitted that intelligence and education tend to parallel health status. If, then, each man finds "good health" a difficult goal, how much more difficult it is for the nurse to help him reach it; she must, in a sense, get "inside the skin" of each of her patients in order to know what he needs. She is temporarily the consciousness of the unconscious, the love of life for the suicidal, the leg of the amputee, the eyes of the newly blind, a means of locomotion for the infant, knowledge and confidence for the young mother, the mouthpiece for those too weak or withdrawn to speak, and so on.

While the nature of nursing partakes of the traditional and timeless values so crucial to care, the contemporary trend toward expanding the scope of nursing practice has offered the public, the legislators, and the professionals some new viewpoints on nursing's potential. Combining highly skilled decision-making and professional accountability to patients, nurse practitioners and clinical specialists in nursing are demonstrating their power and potential to care for people in illness and wellness as independent nursing professionals. As interdependent health workers, sharing cooperatively with others the responsibilities in the delivery of comprehensive health services, these professional nurses add a significant parameter to the present limited medical systems of care. One astute economist voices the opinion that "many individuals overrate the importance of medical care to good health and underrate the importance of nonmedical factors and their own efforts to maintain health."[5]

The characteristic aspects of contemporary nursing may be

conceptualized as follows: (1) Clinical: The major component of clinical care is providing direct care to people. Clinical data must be gathered by qualified nurses at the patient's side. (2) Accountability: Decision-making and accountability are also care, and they are patient-oriented. The nurse practitioner is responsible to the client or the patient. She is not responsible to the physician except as a colleague or team member in that relationship. (3) Collaborative: Some responsibilities are shared and are collaborative. While the nurse practitioner is independent in nursing practice, she interdependently functions in providing care across the spectrum of health and illness in appropriate relationships with other personnel. (4) Health-focused: Care is not illness-oriented. Dis-ease, not disease, is the nurse's major concern. Her goals are to help people to cope with the functions of daily living (exercise, sleep, personal hygiene, nutrition, dental and mental health, relationships with others, etc), despite disabilities, and to help them maintain their wellness. (5) Investigative: Nurse practitioners make multiple observations and investigations of clinical phenomena that will help to improve practice. (6) Change agentry: New patterns for delivery of health care and new ideas for support of the patient's environment and equipment by persons other than nurses are paramount to nursing practice in all parts of the health care system. In this regard, nurse practitioners have had an appreciable influence on the delivery system. (7) Scope of care: The most important aspect of all is that role expansion is increasing the scope of nursing practice, but not changing the nature of practice. This role expansion is designed to expand care. But perhaps a few Venn diagrams with examples will make clear these characteristics. All but the last (Fig. 7) of these have been developed by Dr. Barbara Bates, our medical colleague and staunch supporter of nursing at the University of Rochester Medical Center.

To identify and understand the scope and nature of one's field of practice, it is sometimes fruitful to compare and contrast one's role with the roles of others. Dr. Bates' diagrams help to clarify those relationships.

Figure 1 orients the viewer to the diagrammatic scheme and symbols, with the professional roles designated by a circle in the square of health needs. In Figure 2, medicine's role as well as the roles of many other health professionals are depicted. Note the overlapping of roles and also the unmet health needs that exist despite the multiplicity of roles. For purposes of this discussion, the roles of medicine and nursing are framed in Figure 3. Note the areas of

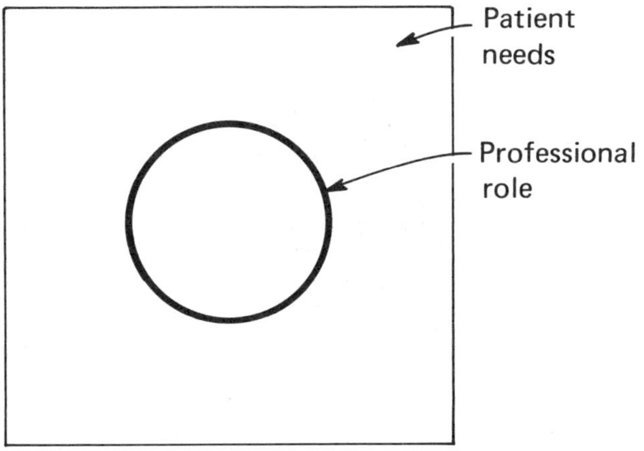

FIG. 1. Patient needs and professional role. (Courtesy of Dr. Barbara Bates.)

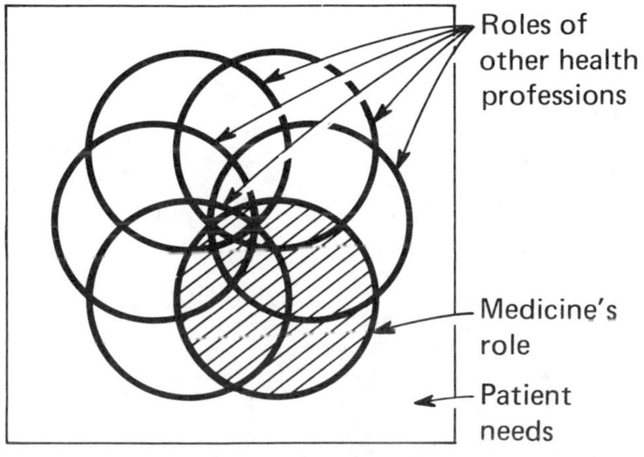

FIG. 2. Medicine and other roles. (Courtesy of Dr. Barbara Bates.)

shared functions and responsibilities. These areas are qualified in Figure 4. Nursing has its major autonomous role in caring, comfort, guiding, and helping. The physician's major role is in diagnosis and treatment. Shared tasks are both instrumental and psychosocial in nature. Role interrelationships are depicted in Figure 5, in which other health workers in areas of nursing and medicine have been added.

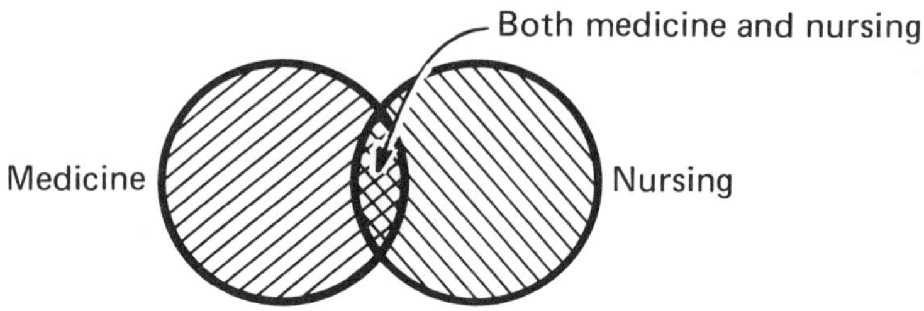

FIG. 3. Roles of medicine and nursing. (Courtesy of Dr. Barbara Bates.)

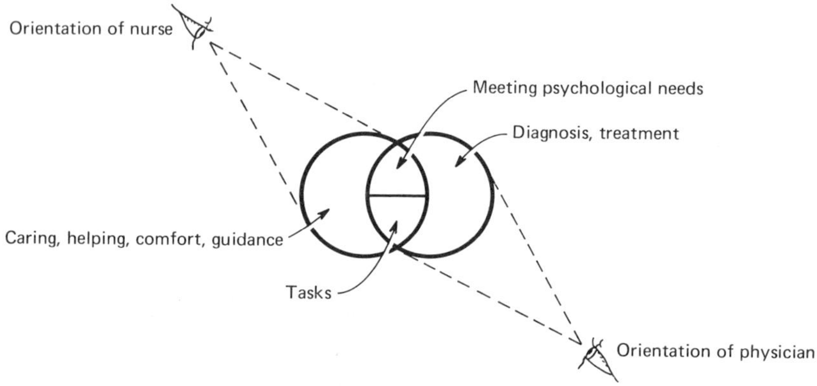

FIG. 4. Roles of medicine and nursing. (Courtesy of Dr. Barbara Bates.)

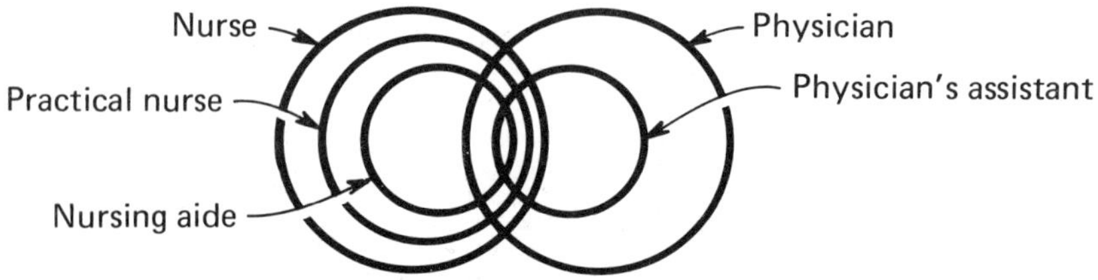

FIG. 5. Role interrelationships. (Courtesy of Dr. Barbara Bates.)

Using that basic orientation to the various relationships, look at the nurse practitioner role in Figure 6, and then extend your thinking about this role as one in which the nurse's expanded role includes serving unmet needs—the needs not met by any worker in the health care system today (Fig. 7). Noticeable gaps, particularly those related to health maintenance services and preventive

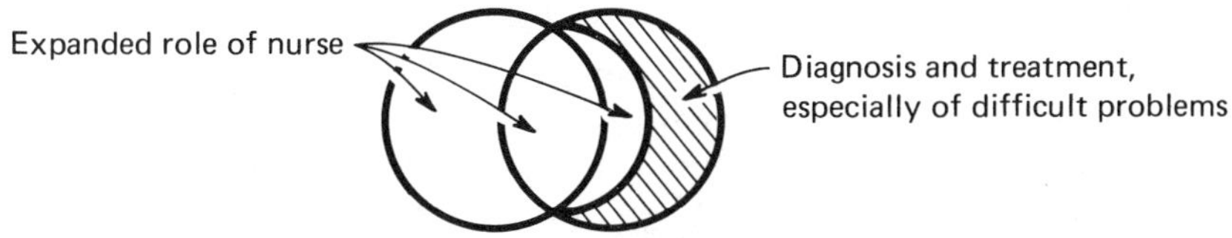

FIG. 6. Expansion of nursing into medicine.

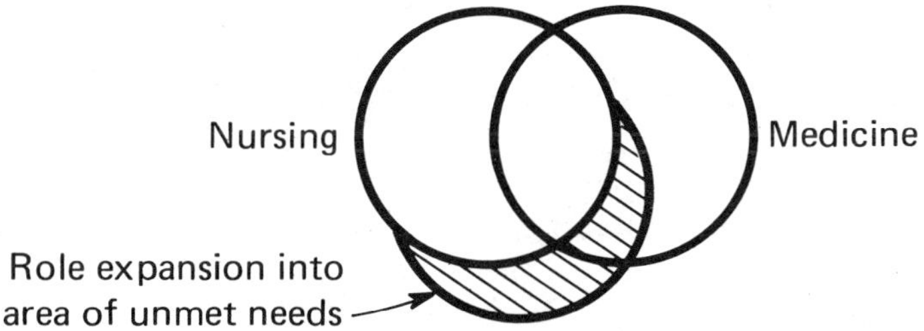

FIG. 7. Expanded role of nurse, including unmet health needs. (Courtesy of Loretta C. Ford, R.N.)

measures, are highly appropriate areas for nursing's attention and concern.

Note that the scope of practice is altered, and indeed it must constantly be in a dynamic state if we are to survive; but note also that the nature of nursing depicted so beautifully by both Nightingale[6] and Henderson[4] remains timeless.

It is from these conceptualizations about the scope and nature of nursing that the standards of quality assurance are constructed. From an understanding of the nature of nursing and nursing roles, some nurses today are working diligently to codify patient responses into nursing diagnoses.

NURSING DIAGNOSES

Efforts to develop a classification system for nursing diagnoses, to identify symptoms and signs of patient responses, and to design effective nursing intervention are under way at the St. Louis University School of Nursing and Allied Health Professions. The stated mission to describe the entire domain of nursing is a monumental task. Further clarification is offered by Gebbie and Lavin:

> This does not mean the identification of all of the tasks performed by nurses or of all the things nurses have ever done in any situation or under any circumstances. These diagnoses focus mainly on the broad health needs of people. The interpretation and resolution of these needs . . . can only be addressed by nurses. What we seek is the identification of these patient problems or concerns most frequently identified by nurses, problems that are usually listed by nurses before they are recognized by other health care workers and problems that are amenable to some intervention . . . available in the present or potential scope of nursing practice.[7]

At the first conference nurses provided a tentative list of nursing diagnoses; here are some samples: alterations in relationships, self-concept, faith, and anxiety and comfort levels; impairments of digestion, family adjustment, and level of consciousness; malnutrition, impaired mobility; pain; sensory disturbances; ineffective sleep and rest patterns; and impairment of verbal communication.[8] These early labels require explication through stated characteristics (signs and symptoms) and subsequent effective nursing intervention, followed by evaluation of outcome; later they may have great usefulness in prediction.

Following the first conference, a Task Force on Modus Operandi was established and charged with the responsibility to identify and execute any activities that could further the goals of the conference, namely identification of those health states diagnosed primarily by nurses, development of a nomenclature for labeling those diagnoses, and development of a system for classifying the identified and labeled problems. Data were requested from 33 institutions on 25 patients in a 30-day collection period. The process of analysis will be facilitated by transferring the diagnostic label, the vital statistics, and patient symptomatology to separate cards from which grouping can be made by a panel of nurse experts.[8] This pilot project will be expanded, if it receives funding, to a 5-year cooperative study on a national plan to make explicit nursing diagnoses and test nursing interventions.

What would this mean for patient care through nursing practice? I believe nurses must increase their communication with each other, with consumers, and with health care team members. Further, nurses must develop investigatory clinical methodologies to demonstrate that nursing care can make a difference. It is hoped that the study will show what those differences are and will show the value of the nursing effort in terms of the health status of patients, in terms of improved reordering of priorities and change in delivery patterns, and in terms of control of the escalating costs of care.

ISSUES IN HEALTH CARE

It is apparent that the cost of medical care, more than any other consideration, has influenced the institution of legislative controls. Many lawmakers believe that current expenditures for all health care are close to the maximum this country is willing to afford; pouring more financial resources into the present system will not redirect the allocations or correct imbalances.

In 1972, expenditures for health care were $90 billion; in 1973 they were $94 billion. It is estimated that by 1976 the national health expenditures will exceed $110 billion, and projections for 1980 range between $155 billion and $190 billion.[9] In analyzing health care and the economic system in the United States, health economist Victor Fuchs has said that there are two fallacies that obstruct our thinking.[9] One is that resources are no longer scarce, and the other is that health is the most important goal nationally. Fuchs substantiates his claim by example of the choices that will have to be made between alternatives. All the other decisions that people make daily about their health make it clear that they frequently place a higher value on satisfying other wants, eg, smoking, overeating, careless driving, and failure to take medicine.[9]

However, unless health care can be differentiated from medical care and a clear enunciation made of a social policy for health, few, if any, major changes will be made in the allocation of national resources for health care.

Equating health with medicine makes health a medical problem—not a social problem, and not even the consumer's problem. From such a spurious equation, territoriality with its strong professional, political, economic, and social barriers becomes established. Larger health-related social problems such as poverty, aging, nutrition, housing, and environmental pollution are being ignored. Resource allocations for medical services become skewed to favor advancing ideas and technology for acute care to the neglect of basic research, preventive measures, rehabilitation, and support for care other than medical care.[10] There exists a monolithic system dedicated to searching out pathology in individuals. Further, a system that is controlled by one provider of services (the medical establishment) has resulted. A minority of medical providers called physicians, some 330,000 strong, controls access to all the health care delivered by the 4.5 million health workers (75 percent of whom are women) to the nation's 215 million people.

Conceptualizing health in the broadest social terms will require not only reform of political and economic systems but also reorientation of professional interests and consideration of emerging consumer needs and expectations. There is also the need to think of the organization of care in new ways. Garfield has devised some ideas about availability and costs through the Kaiser Health Insurance Plan. Diagrammatic representations (Figs. 8 and 9) show the growing complexities of technologic development from 1900, the growing demand for health care for all people, and the concept of a health maintenance organization (Fig. 10) in which subscribers to a

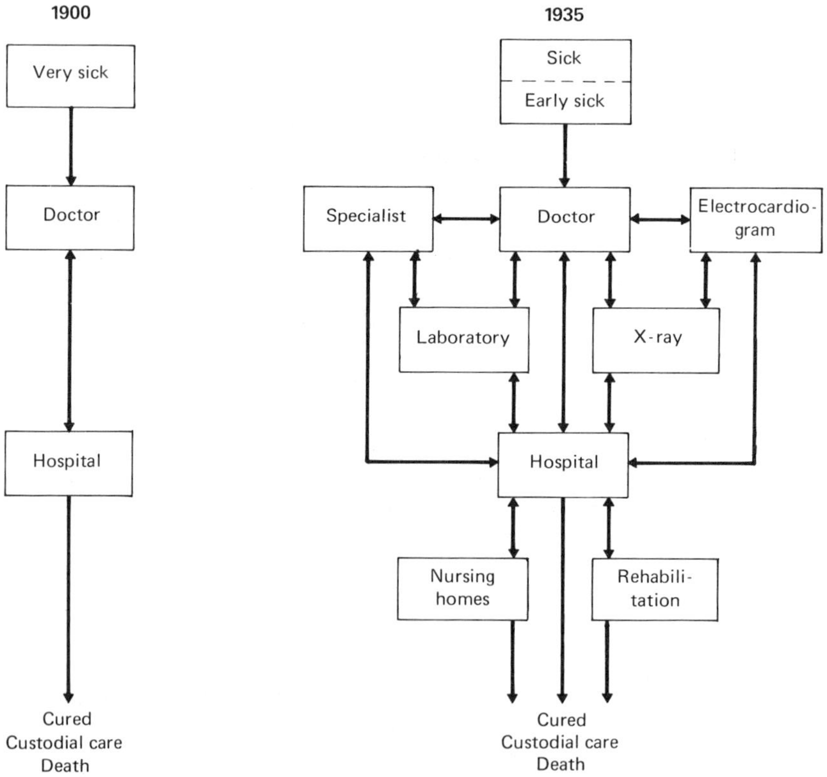

FIG. 8. Growing complexity of technologic development. (Source: Sidney R. Garfield, "The Delivery of Medical Care," *Scientific American*, 222: 15-23 (p. 21), April, 1970.)

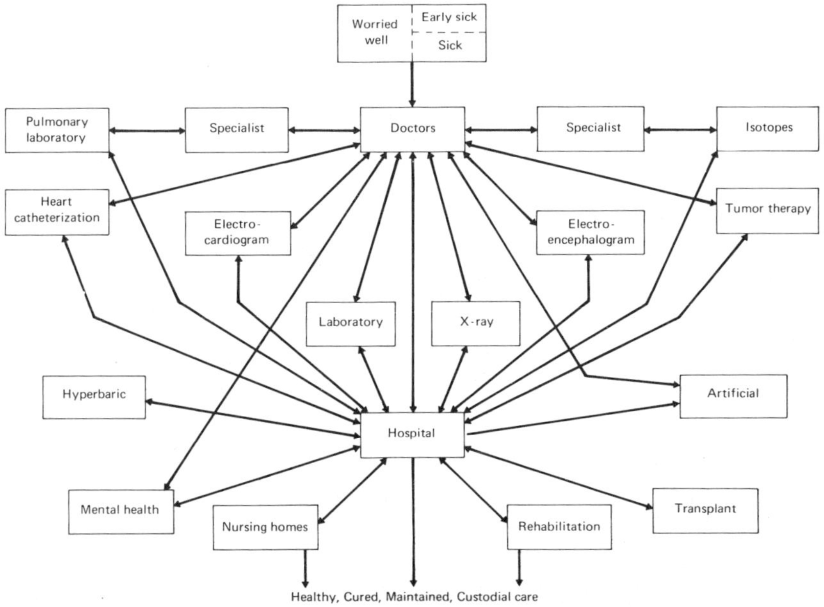

FIG. 9. Growing demand for health care. (Source: Sidney R. Garfield, "The Delivery of Medical Care," *Scientific American*, 222: 15-23 (p. 21), April, 1970.)

health care plan are active participants in a comprehensive family prepaid insurance plan. In this latter type of service the focus is on maintaining the wellness of the subscribers; the plan provides the incentive of lower premiums to the subscriber and also rewards the provider financially.

OPTIONS, RISKS, AND GUIDELINES

One might wonder what all this has to do with independent practice in nursing. The obvious implication is that the general movement in health care financing is away from fee for service to prepayment plans with increasing governmental controls. While I believe that nurses could inaugurate health maintenance organizations offering consumers comprehensive health care by using nurse practitioners and clinical specialists, and contracting with physicians and other health workers to provide their particular kinds of care, I know of no independent nurse practitioners who are considering such an enterprise.

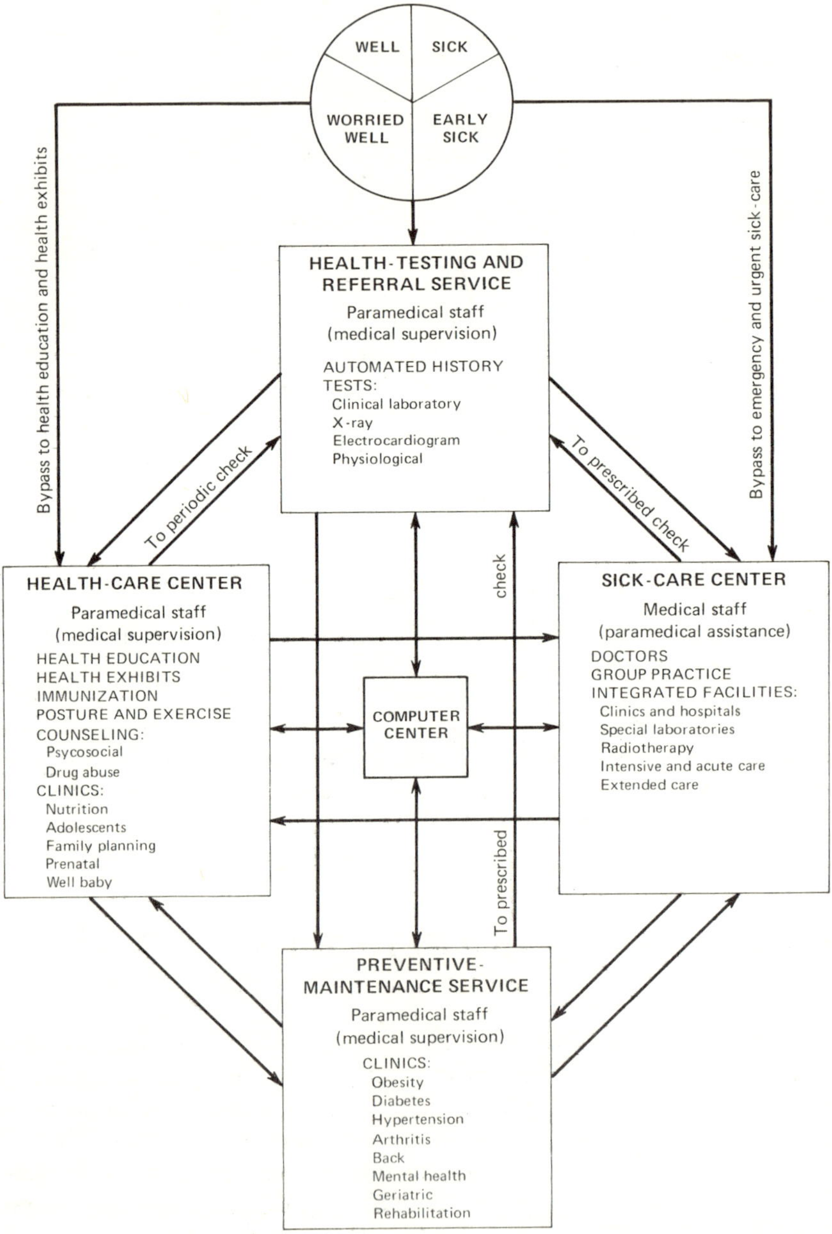

FIG. 10. Health maintenance organization. (Source: Sidney R. Garfield, "The Delivery of Medical Care," *Scientific American*, 222, 15-23 (p. 21), April, 1970.)

Perhaps it is too much to ask that nurses (99 percent of whom are women) should initiate bold, risky plans to be the prime deliverers of health care. Despite the fact that 75 percent of the health workforce is female, few positions of power at the political or professional levels are held by women. This is true in all countries of the world, not just the United States. For example, although a large percentage of medical doctors in the Soviet Union are women, male physicians hold the prestigious directorships of institutes, hospitals, etc. However, the developments of recent years offer new hope that women and nurses will seize the increasing opportunities for leadership in health care policy and organizational development. The big question is this: Are women (and nurses) prepared to assume and willing to assume such roles? Are there statespersons among nurses with the vision and wisdom to lead the way? Certainly those of you in independent professional practice have demonstrated a willingness to take risks for yourselves. But is that enough? Are you willing to transfer that courage to a larger mission? Can you afford, now that you are private entrepreneurs, to address broader national issues? Who will mind the store while you contribute to the national effort? Women are caught up in a worldwide phenomenon of social change that is often uncertain, fast-paced, and complex. Esther Lucille Brown often says, "Nurses think change is an event rather than a process." Change is indeed a process, with phases, probabilities, and predictabilities that any astute change agent knows. I imagine that all of you have discovered that and have worked out for yourselves the strategies, logistics, and tactics to deal with change. It is to be hoped that you've also discovered some survival skills. For me, those skills come through theoretical formulations about change from which understandings are gleaned and strategies are devised. A few suggestions might help:

1. Find joy in risk-taking and change. The stresses of change can be exhilarating if you don't take yourself or others too seriously.
2. Maintain a high tolerance for ambiguities. In times of rapid change there are few stable situations. Expecting or creating a great deal of structure is unrealistic and often detrimental to the change process.
3. Permit yourself the right to fail. From failure you can learn a great deal about yourself and others; so don't be afraid to take risks or admit failure. Use the experience as a learning adventure.
4. Learn the name and rules of the game. If you engage in a war, be able to distinguish between a skirmish and a battle, and behave accordingly.

5. Devise your own support system outside the system you're trying to change. Everybody needs to feel wanted and loved, but change agents seldom are loved in the system they seek to change. You'll need a personal support system all your own.

6. Despite all failures and frustrations, remember the sun will come up tomorrow; so you'll have a whole new day to start over. Being in the forefront of carving out new directions can be a rewarding, exciting, and frustrating experience. Why not give it a whirl?

REFERENCES

1. Health Planning and Resources Development Act of 1974. U.S. Department of Health, Education, and Welfare. Public Health Service. Health Resources Administration, Bureau of Health Planning and Resources Development. DHEW Publication (HRA) 75–14015.
2. Hall VC: Statutory Regulation of the Scope of Nursing Practice—A Critical Survey. 1975. National Joint Practice Commission, 875 N. Michigan Avenue, Suite 1864, John Hancock Center. Chicago, Ill, 60611
3. New York Education Law 6902, 1972
4. Henderson VA: The Nature of Nursing. New York, Macmillan, 1966.
5. Campbell RR: Economics of Health and Public Policy. Washington DC, American Enterprise Institute, 1971
6. Nightingale F: Notes on Nursing. London, Duckworth, 1952 (First published in 1859)
7. Gebbie K, Lavin MA: Classification of nursing diagnosis. Am J Nurs 70:250, 1974
8. St Louis University Research Report No. 1. August 1974
9. Fuchs V: Socioeconomic Issues in Health. Chicago, AMA, 1974
10. Birenbaum A: The making of a professional identity: the pediatric nurse practitioner. Journal of Voluntary Action Research 3: Summer 1974, p 98

SECTION II

PRACTICE AND BEYOND

CHAPTER 8

Defining Nursing: A Haunting Refrain

For over 100 years nursing has been preoccupied with defining itself. As nursing has become more complex, it has become increasingly difficult to formulate a short statement comprehensive enough to encompass the depth and scope of nursing practice. Considerable effort has also gone into attempts to define nursing practice at its various levels: unskilled, technical, and professional. In the last few years there has been a moratorium on this obsession of defining, and nurses have found some comfort in the recognition that there are many definitions of nursing, depending on health needs to be met, area of clinical specialization, interest in various aspects of practice, and context in which nursing practice is carried on.

RECOGNITION WITHIN THE HEALTH CARE SYSTEM

It appears that in terms of the health care sytem, nursing is once again at a point of crisis. Without a definition, there is a threat to its survival. National health insurance is coming closer to realization. At any given time at least half a dozen national health insurance bills are pending. This legislation will identify health care givers and what health care givers will be permitted to do and will be restricted from doing. It is appalling to think that there are bills among the proposed legislation that have written nursing out—national health insurance with nurses written out, models of health centers without nurses involved, and insurance companies developing third-party payment policy for everyone but nurses. If these proposals become law they could wipe out the profession. Every group giving health care needs recognition in order to survive in the face of the tremendous social change now in progress.

COMPETITION FOR POWER IN THE HEALTH CARE SYSTEM

Other health professionals tend to ignore or deny what they do not want to hear from nurses. This is not new to nursing, but it may increase as the pace of competition increases. Gertrude Isaacs makes this comment:

> As long ago as 1932, on the basis of studies of the practices of nurses–midwives at the Frontier Nursing Service in Hyden, Kentucky, there was evidence that a similar care system for the whole country would reduce maternal mortality by 10,000 deaths per year and prevent 30,000 stillborn deliveries and newborn deaths. Until very recently nurse midwifery as an alternative to medical obstetrics for maternity care has been largely ignored, even for rural and other populations deprived of skilled obstetric care. It is still more popular with the consumer than with physicians.

Longitudinal studies involving hundreds of thousands of visits of nurses to patients and clients have yielded evidence that nurses can provide care that is comparable to or superior to that of physicians, particularly in chronic illness.[1-3] Other short and poorly controlled studies published in prestigious medical journals report the opposite.[4-7] In some studies the failure of nurses in the areas studied appears to have been designed into the study. Many physicians feel threatened by nurses who practice independently and are fully accountable for their practice.

The recently published *Selected Bibliography with Abstracts in Joint Practice* prepared by the National Joint Practice Commission,[8] while using terminology about joint practice that is acceptable to nurses and calling nurses physicians' associates (rather than assistants), insinuates the basic message that nurses must be supervised by physicians and that they are really employees. This kind of approach may be as effective a tool for consolidating power as ignoring and contradicting research findings about nurse practitioners. Successful competition for a place in the health care system is not possible without an accepted statement of identifiable services.

RESISTANCE TO CHANGE IN THE HEALTH CARE BUREAUCRACY

An increase in the number of nurses competent in generalized ambulatory care is sure to reduce the number of hospitalizations. This may be one of nursing's greatest social and economic contributions to health care. But we have expensive hospital complexes. We have a huge bureaucracy selling insurance to pay hospital, not ambulatory care, bills. Do hospital administrators and Blue Cross/Blue Shield want to hear that nurses can reduce hospitalization for patients over 65 years of age by 25 percent? Do hospital administrators want to cut down on the use of hospital beds when many are hardly at the break-even point now? Does Blue Cross/Blue Shield, so closely allied with the growth of hospitals, want to make the great modification of paying for all ambulatory health care? No! The system requires that inpatient days be kept high. Blue Cross/Blue Shield wants to know the cost benefits; nursing costs may be higher, but the social value of the care may also be higher. Utilization review may now support keeping hospital beds occupied rather than identifying preventable illness or nonhospital resources for care. We are beginning to get some hard data in this area; eg, Ralph Nader's health research group indicated that there is a surplus of 100,000 hospital beds in the United States and 250,000 that are being underused.[9] But strong institutionalized forces operate to maintain the existing system and the definition of nursing that supports the system. Definition of nursing is critical to modification of the health care delivery system.

COMPETITION FOR ROLE AND FUNCTION IN THE HEALTH CARE SYSTEM

The struggle going on for nursing's right to a position on the health care team, a share in comprehensive health care, and the right to do independent work with clients is a basic reason for making more explicit the definition of nursing. In psychiatry, particularly, the struggle is critical. Recently the American Psychiatric Association appealed to third-party payer insurance companies to make sure that when they pay for psychotherapy it is medical psychotherapy. But insurance companies have been heavily pressured by the American Psychological Association, the American Nurses Association, and the National Association of Social Workers to decide that psychotherapy not be defined strictly as medical psychotherapy. This situation has arisen not only because of competition from emerging groups of nonmedical psychotherapists but also because some physicians have been slow to give up the long and tedious psychoanalytic approach to treatment and have thus lost community support. The field of psychiatry will be increasingly competitive. Third-party payers are saying: Why should we pay you at the rate of $35 per hour when the psychologist is also doing this? Nurses must also present their services from the best vantage point, so that the contribution they can make will be seen to be as beneficial as the contributions of others.

Maddy Gerrish described how the lack of nursing definition and lack of profession support for it affected her:

> I practice in Massachusetts and have had a part-time private practice since 1963. In 1973, I formed a corporation, Expansion Inc., to practice. At about the same time there was great concern on the part of the Board of Psychology in Massachusetts that various people were delivering psychological services without having the credentials to do so. This was followed by the movement to restrict non-credentialed people from practicing.
>
> Nursing stayed out of this movement, both at the state nursing level and the Board of Registration. It was an unfortunate decision. As a result of that action the Board of Psychology in Massachusetts in conjunction with state legislation passed a law stating that anyone who delivers psychological services in the state must be either licensed as a psychologist or supervised by a licensed psychologist or a psychiatrist. I chose to get licensed as a psychologist so that I could retain the directorship of Expansion and maintain my integrity as supervisor of this organization. All of my credentials are in psychiatric nursing, yet I would be forced to have supervision in nursing from a psychologist or psychiatrist. The nurse practice law meant absolutely nothing in Massachusetts.

Not only must nurses either give nursing a better identity or become lost in psychology or sociology or treatments and procedures, they must also become fully aware of what is going on and promote an active role for nursing in the political arena. Such compromises cannot be made by all nurses and should not have to be made by all. But what are the alternatives until nursing can be redefined as a function other than an extension of other disciplines?

EQUITABLE REDISTRIBUTION OF NURSES

Status, role, and function as parts of a definition of nursing must be formalized and linked up with a legal position. Section D, the miscellaneous part of the new Nurse Training and Education Act,[10] requires that procedures as yet unspecified are to be set up and used by the secretary of the Department of Health, Education, and Welfare to count nurses, state by state, and to decide whether there is an undersupply, an adequate supply, or an oversupply. Then legislation will be introduced that will tie support of nursing education to equitable redistribution of nurses. Local physicians may be given the authority and be made responsible for health care unless there is some kind of linkage to a nationally accepted legal or official nursing definition or position. Nursing stands to lose what autonomy it has, in addition to having to be concerned about distributing people to places comparable to those where they currently work. This is going to happen, and it threatens to happen so fast that nursing will not have a voice in developing plans and will not be ready to plug into emerging models of health care.

GUIDE TO CHANGING NURSING PRACTICE ACTS AND ACTION BY ORGANIZED NURSING

In almost all the states where nursing practice acts have recently been changed, nursing has in some respects been set back 20 years by statements about nursing practice that attempt to make nursing an extension of another profession. An extensive study by Kissam documents this.[11] These statements indicate that nursing is permitted or allowed independent functions and dependent functions. One profession cannot be allowed functions or be supervised by another profession. To the extent that dependent functions are spelled out, the nursing license is worthless, since it is the physician's license the nurse is working under and medical care she is doing. Among some nurses, there is a sense of urgency to identify nursing as an independent profession. Since most nurses do not feel comfortable unless they are tied to another profession or to a responsible institution, most of the work done on the nursing practice laws spells out medical care functions; but this work is peripheral to the core of nursing, and these revisions do not deal with the main problem. Once again nursing seems to be letting external events influence the determination of what nursing is. Nurses need to eliminate outside influences, study their practice, document it, relate it to a theoretical framework, revise and modify both practice and framework until they feel secure in their practice, and know that they are practicing nursing.

COMMUNICATION AMONG NURSES

It is a false assumption that in any relationship among nurses, whether in individual relationships or in organized meetings, they are talking about the same thing when they use the word nursing. To provide for any common ground and unity of purpose, there must be a new definition that is accepted throughout the profession.

PUTTING AN END TO DEFINITION BY OTHERS

Nurses have commonly looked to other people for assistance in defining themselves—physicians, social scientists, hospital administrators, academicians, patients, and clients. Nursing should mature and produce clinical leadership so that practicing nurses and their clients can define the professional practice of nursing. One problem in defining nursing is that if psychiatric nursing or midwifery should become known as the function that constitutes nursing, and if all nurses cannot do what these nurses do (in their capacity as scientific and medical functionaries), then those who cannot do these things will not meet the requirements of nursing or of being a nurse. Will not all the specialties (which are offshoots of medical specialties) leave nursing fragmented and nurses divided group against group? This is the plight of the generalist. Generalists don't practice psychology or psychiatry. They are not "scopers and thumpers." Generalists have considerable difficulty in defining nursing. When asked what they do, they may say, "I do what has to be done." But they have never conceptualized or documented what it is or how it is unique to nursing, ie, it cannot be done by other health care givers.

More than ever before, medicine is working to move nursing into the area of medical practice. Lucille Kinlein provides a case in point with coronary care:

> As scientific technology improved, patients in coronary care units needed skilled medical care around the clock. Physicians chose the most intelligent young nurses and trained them to give medical care and function as doctor substitutes. Nurses responded and abdicated their nursing care roles in favor of carrying out what was identified as nursing by the medical profession. What goes on in most coronary care units is not nursing. Supervisors and directors of nursing are caught up in this. The nurse can neglect the patient's family, neglect to support him emotionally, neglect his comfort, privacy, modesty needs, and the like, and no one notices, but let her not give medication on time or miss a slight aberration in the cardiogram and she is taken to task. Reports on nursing care in coronary care units are limited, and statistics reporting the effectiveness of these units are medical statistics, not nursing statistics. Nurses have no quarrel with the nurse being in the coronary care unit, because it saves lives, but it replaces the spirit of nursing with the mechanics of nursing.

DEFINING NURSING IS NOT IMPORTANT

Of what importance is it that what the nurse does is defined? Except for pregnancy and childbirth, it is deviation from the normal or discovery of pathology that brings people into the health care system. This fact determines interdisciplinary aspects of primary care. What is important is not what nursing is, but that people are getting the primary care they need and never had before. Many people think that it makes no sense to define nursing because today there is a team approach to care. What is really important is what works and why. It does not matter that there is considerable role overlap among disciplines.

As an example, the Emory University School of Nursing developed a new nursing service. They have a contract to provide primary care to a liberal arts college student population. They have a medical backup panel, but they are not forcing a distinction between what is nursing and what is doctoring. College health services, especially services to this age group, are usually very negative, but the feedback about this program from students is exceptionally positive. People are finding they can get things they could not get before. Everyone is surprised that it is working so well. One of the key aspects seems to be that they are not making a clear differentiation between nursing and medicine. They consult with physicians about the performance of certain medical acts, with physician backup. They have a system.

Another important argument for leaving nursing undefined is reduction of interprofessional conflict and intraprofessional conflict and avoidance of alienation of the specialized groups of nurses from their colleagues. The time for activism in regard to role definition will come once the skills are learned and are taught to a new generation of nurses, once nurses have some consensus on which piece of the health care pie they wish to claim and struggle for.

EXCERPTS FROM DISCUSSION

One point I always feel a great urgency to make is that nursing is an independent profession. Nursing is geared to wellness, as opposed to illness, and while I have had problems defining both of those concepts, I am definitely able to function in a health-supporting health-promoting role. . . .

My problem is that I feel the nurse definitely has a role, but she can function so much better as a member of a team where they are all together. There are so many things with both wellness and patient illness that I cannot handle alone. But together with other professionals we can really do a great job. I'm thinking of eyes, for example, and all the things that can happen. I think it is an interdependent type of thing more than independent. It takes more than a nurse to keep a person well. It takes more than me and the patients. . . .

One of nursing's primary functions is education toward self-care and self-responsibility for health, and that is independent. Nurses must attempt to work themselves out of a job. . . .

Does any other professional title himself (define himself) as a team member in order to fully practice his profession under his or her license? . . .

Maybe we should differentiate between being on a team and collaborating. Being on a team, to me, means you are all working in the same area, or you all get together to discuss a patient. Collaboration might mean you would not even be in the same physical setting. . . .

Some of the ambiguity arises because no one person is educated to take care of the total needs of an individual. . . .

The nurse is educated to look into a person's health and take care of his health or help him take care of himself. If there is deviation from normal, nurses refer the person for medical care, or it might be social service care. This is where communication comes in. I invite the client to recognize this problem. He, when he recognizes it, may very well decide he can put up with it. I collaborate with him at this time. I help him make an informed choice, but it is his responsibility to decide. This is the essence of what I have to offer. . . .

If we have six nurses who call themselves independent nurse practitioners, then the public has the right to look at what each one of them is doing. The public won't find them doing the same things. Each person must do what the others are doing to be able to call it the independent practice of nursing. This is not related to functions and tasks, but to a concept of nursing that will say to the world at large that there is unanimity about what a nurse in independent practice means to the community. This hasn't been done in any other context of nursing practice; so this compounds a problem that was not dealt with at an earlier time. . . .

As soon as we attach specialization to nursing, we are immediately in another field, another profession. As a medical-surgical nurse with a specialty in cardiovascular nursing, I was not teaching nursing. I was teaching electrophysiology of the myocardium. As soon as you say cardiovascular nursing or psychiatric nursing you are medically oriented to that specialization, and nursing is a second word added to another field. So we are nurses practicing psychiatry, nurses practicing cardiovascular care. . . .

The conflicts between generalists and specialists in defining nursing create division. Generalists demand that everyone be alike, otherwise nursing is fragmented. Specialists won't talk about being fragments of nursing. The kind of revolution you are talking about, as a generalist, is that those of us who practice a speciality are not practicing nursing. You are talking about nursing adhering to a certain philosophy that if followed through would eliminate specialities in nursing.

I would like to suggest a forum for nurses to talk about their nursing care so that we as peers can hear what each is saying and analyze it in light of an operational definition of nursing accepted for the forum. It might be that we could not accept an operational definition until we all present what we think is our nursing care. We should be able to see a core of nursing care, something that becomes nursing. We are not saying that we would push anybody out of nursing. It would allow us to say: This is the core. As you move into a specialty you take that core or some of it with you. . . .

I don't practice psychology. It is peripheral that I am a licensed psychologist. I felt I had to prove that my nursing skills and my nursing credentials would hold up in my state against those of all the other people who were being allowed to practice in the delivery of psychological services. I call myself a nurse. My brochures call me a nurse. But it is a fact that I have to be licensed as a psychologist to offer nursing services. Despite the contradiction, I had to decide what was best, to practice or not to practice and be out of business.

My credentials are in nursing, but I have to compete with other disciplines to deliver psychological services. In this society, I can't say that what I do as a nurse psychotherapist is different from what a psychologist does. I'm different because I'm a person, but I have to compete in the system to get third-party payments as a nurse psychotherapist. The consumer in our society, right now, is saying, "We want certain kinds of services, and we are willing to pay for certain kinds of services." There may be little concern as to who provides the service; what matters is that consumers get the kind and quality of service they want.

PROBLEMS

Two of us, independent nurse practitioners, both generalists, were sitting at a table discussing contractual relations, and we found that we had different conceptions of what independence is, what kinds of contractual arrangements there should be with physicians, or whether we should just go on a referral basis. We couldn't even agree on the extent to which telephone calls obligate one. We finally decided that each had her own style and we wouldn't try to come up with a common style. . . .

We have been discussing nursing roles for years. It is almost as if the role expands and contracts according to how many physicians are in the situation.

This is clearly where, to me, the focus makes all the difference. Part of the reason we have failed to identify nursing to our health professional colleagues is that all the examples of nursing given start with a medically oriented condition. We always start with diabetes, or hypertension, and then we say what we do to prevent hospitalization. What we do is to prevent more complication. This becomes a nurse applying her knowledge to achieve a medical goal.

I don't separate them completely, because I see that health practices are designed to keep you well, but they are also designed to prevent illness. So I can't separate them completely. I see what you mean about health, and it isn't just prevention. It is also promoting good health. We do not have this in the literature to present to the public. . . .

The reality of the health care situation is that illness and medical care have the priority. This is particularly important to nurses where there are few physicians. If there were an adequate number of physicians for illness care, priorities might change for the nurse's clientele to much more of a health maintenance/health education approach. . . .

We in the nursing community have recently agonized over efforts to define ourselves, which has always been impossible. We cannot decide what we are, because our value is determined by the public. That is the place to find the definition of ourselves. And to the extent the public finds value in what we are doing, and we assign a fee structure appropriate for the value, that is our groundwork for professional practice. Knowledge is in the task. We are never going to define it. . . .

The ICN has a definition of nursing. Will you buy that? No, because it has not been arrived at logically. The ICN definition is the result of identification of needs flowing from a medically oriented definition of needs. I think the time has come when the only way we are going to define nursing is to hear what each one of us is willing to lay out for all the rest of us to see and treat in analytic fashion. What happened between me and my client I now present to you my colleagues as my nursing care. Critical incidents do not give us nursing care. . . .

Why do we have to use the phrase nurse practitioners? Practitioner is a tautology added to the word nurse. It is more than a semantic problem; it is our unwillingness and inability to accept the intrinsic meaning of the word nurse, which conveys practice.

DEFINITION BY PRACTITIONERS

With or without definition, the nurses in practice provide data about their work. Many of these data are provided in the form of critical incidents and descriptions. While critical incidents and vignettes of practice do not define nursing practice, they point out changes in focus and trends that will be incorporated into the definition of practice. The critical incidents that were contributed indicated concern with health care, advocacy, crisis care, and primary care, as well as illness care. The following examples illustrate this.

Focus on Health

After a year and a half of joint nurse–physician practice, the physician I was working with told me that he thought he understood what the nurse contributes to the patient's care. He said, "The nurse is concerned with health, and as a physician I'm more concerned with disease." I agreed, and we discussed this further. It was a long time coming, but he finally understood what I had said many, many times. . . .

Through consumer education, many people are becoming less crisis-oriented. A person called and informed us that she could not afford our services, but would like some information about her medications and her health in general. She was in her menopausal years and wanted to know what to expect, where she could receive services at a price she could afford, and what the alternatives were if she did not seek care. We have received many telephone calls that were not for illness but for health information. . . .

One patient requested to see her cervix with a mirror. . . .

I have been successful in helping families get their symptomatic kids under control by working only on the parental relationship. . . .

I was called for counseling by a 22-year-old woman who had been in a previous awareness group. She said she could not pay the minimum on the sliding-fee scale of $15 per hour. I suggested other agencies, but as we talked we realized that I already knew her (eliminating reiteration of any history) and that she was familiar with my therapy approach and only needed some support and specific application with my help. We agreed that a maximum of two sessions was necessary (at $10 per hour, which she could afford). She wanted an appointment that day; so we met after her work. It turned out that some simple problem-solving—a wider range of choices—was the only need. She had been coping extremely well with a complete new life style brought about by a weight loss of 80 pounds. She had lived as a "fatty" until the previous year and had then become slim and beautiful. Her one area of confusion was with her sexual behavior with males. She had met a man with whom she thought she might become friendly, but she was concerned about her appearance nude if they went to bed. She had loose flesh on her abdomen that was to be removed surgically at a later date. We discussed the choices of behavior that she might make, and she felt more confident. She was also reassured about her own sexuality by our discussion, because she had had a same-sex relationship about which she had told no one else. . . .

I'm working to support people's ability and to meet their needs to survive. . . .

We are applying some really good theory to life style change and threat prevention, advocacy, and planning for fixed-income living. What happens to the survivor when one spouse dies? People come who have been the rounds of specialists and don't know what it all means. They want to know, they want it explained—not be talked down. . . .

We knew it was going to take time to educate the public as to what we were there for, and we found in 2 years that we didn't know what the public wanted from us. Now we know what people are coming for. We are also very humble about what we call these things. They are not coming to us because they know they need preoperation preparation, for example; they are coming because they want certain kinds of information and assistance. If we have a name for it, in the marketing sense, we can say, "We've got this." It relates to what you could call the important dimensions. So we are moving into the marketing mode to find out from the consumer what it is. . . .

I support a nurse friend at Planned Parenthood, and she provides my referred clients with the best services her agency offers. I tell her what clients tell me they need, and she, being assistant director, often institutes new services to meet client needs. For example, I suggested that clinic nurses fit diaphragms. The agency trained nurses to do that. I have also suggested that women over 40 years of age have many needs related to their reproductive systems. Now PP is beginning to provide new services for this neglected group. We have discussed therapy ideas also, and she has adapted my concept to her clients and co-workers. . . .

I don't want to be a "junior doctor." I want to offer nursing services the patient might not get otherwise: teaching, counseling, listening. . . .

During our mass hypertension screening program in a pharmacy, many of the people who came in for blood pressure checks took the opportunity to talk about other things such as side effects of medication, particularly impotence with many of the antihypertensives—symptoms that led us to make referrals to the local free clinic, health department, and Planned Parenthood. Women needed to talk about their children or husbands or jobs, and they were surprised to learn that there were agencies that could help them when we made referrals. People will talk to health professionals if we will listen and sit still long enough. Pharmacies are an excellent place to provide this listening, teaching, and referral. . . .

Mrs. K. is in her middle 70s; she is Jewish, and she came to the United States from Vienna during World War II. She came via concentration camps and still has the tattoo as a visible reminder of the horrors she cannot forget. Her daughter, who also lives in the county, is her only relative. The daughter does not understand her mother and never has. Mrs. K. cannot talk to either her or to her friends comfortably. So at periodic intervals, as she chooses, she comes in and talks to me about Vienna, the war, the horrors, her loneliness, her boredom with the activities at the local temple, her longing for prewar Vienna. She cries sometimes and kisses me on the cheek when she leaves. . . .

Two sisters who live together come in regularly. Both are in their 70s. T.

has never married, and she retired from a fascinating job after 30 years—at 52 years of age. Since then she has traveled and generally had a ball on her substantial pension. Her sister G. is a widow with two daughters who live within 100 miles. G.'s income is limited basically to Social Security; so she lives with T. The daughters are very grateful to their aunt T. for agreeing to live with G. At first T. was terribly upset with the situation. She said, "G. always was bossy!" Now she has accepted the reality of their living situation and has resumed her old activities, even though G. does not often participate. G. has become increasingly depressed of late, saying, "I really don't care what happens to me any more." G. is gaining weight, and her blood pressure continues to be elevated, even though she is on medication, which she takes. T.'s blood pressure, also treated, is controlled, and she is losing weight. We see them separately, and each has a chance to talk about the other as well as herself. Our experience with making referrals to anything remotely related to mental health for clients like G. results in comments such as, "Oh, so you think I'm crazy." Often that's the last we see of them. As a result, we continue to provide listening and counseling services, seeking case-based consultation from colleages in psychiatric–mental health nursing as needed. Occasionally one of our mental health colleagues does see clients, providing us with opportunities both to observe and to be observed in counseling. . . .

Mrs. C., 63 years of age, a married, recently retired teacher, came into the pharmacy to have her blood pressure checked. She came in response to the poster in the pharmacy window. She had discontinued all of her medications and was attempting to "clear the chemicals out of her system." As we talked it became clear that she was profoundly depressed; she was upset about her relationship with her husband, her lack of interest in life, her decreasing contacts with outsiders, her diminishing level of physical activity—all of which she mourned but could not counteract. After suggesting a variety of activities, which she invariably dismissed for some reason or another, I finally pointed out that she was playing the "Yes, but. . . ." game with whatever we talked about. What, I asked, did she think she wanted to do about her situation? She proposed that about the only thing she could do at the time was to resume her regular walks. I discussed some of the advantages such as increased oxygenation that such activity might bring. She described the length of walk she felt she could manage, and I wrote up a short contract statement. She was very surprised when I asked her to sign the contract to take a walk every day for a week. She did initial it after further discussion. An hour later as I drove home from the pharmacy, I saw her striding back toward her home, head down, frowning, but walking! The next week she came back in to report, tersely, that she had indeed walked every day. She signed another contract for the next week. She telephoned to say that she had continued walking and was beginning to lose some weight. On a recent visit she was still off all medications; she had bought an exercise bicycle and was experimenting with natural foods. She started on kelp because someone told her it was a good source of iron. She was astounded when we looked kelp up and discovered that kelp is high in sodium and low in iron. Her expression is still dour, but she admits that her moods are less disastrous than before. . . .

Advocacy

Quite often the pharmacist in our area forgets to label medications with the name of the drug. Once he dispensed digoxin and phenobarbital to a client in similar vials. Both medications were to be taken twice daily. Because of some unforeseen situation, the person's physician increased one of the medications to four times a day. Since the medications looked alike, the person did not know which to take four times a day. We spoke with the pharmacist, and since this incident our clients' medications have been labeled correctly. Several pharmacists were involved in our discussion of the consumer's right to competent services. . . .

An elderly couple use our services in their planning for disability or for the death of one, which would leave the other in need of some advocacy in the health care system. Should the wife die first, we are prepared to provide the husband with continuity of advocacy from knowledge and documentation of life style, functional capabilities, preferences, and medical history. . . .

When one of our clients is hospitalized, we see him in the hospital in an effort to maintain continuity of care. We share our information with other professional groups, including nurses, social workers, dieticians, physicians, and clergymen. In several instances we did not have to seek permission to read our clients' hospital records; instead, their records have been shared with us. Clergymen and nurses have sought our advice in meeting our clients' needs. Further, nurses have informed us of the dates our clients were expected to return to their families and their communities. . . .

When we and our pharmacist colleagues began planning to put on hypertension screening programs in local pharmacies, we invited some of the local physicians to join us at our breakfast meetings. We already had much of the mechanics worked out, but we needed physician input on what to consider abnormal blood pressures, and more important we needed them to accept referrals should we find someone in need of immediate medical care who either had no physician or whose physician was away. All went along well until we said that we were going to explain what blood pressure is and does and give each client a written copy of his reading. The doctors were less than enthusiastic about our giving clients their blood pressure readings. "That will only worry them," we were told. We made it clear that people needed adequate and accurate information on which to base their decisions. Either we were going to give them as much information and as sound information as we could or there would be no program—that was that. We had no problems. People took and continue to take our little slips of paper with blood pressure readings and other written reminders of things we talked about that they might want to talk to their doctors about. We did not go to the medical society to ask them about or tell them about what we're doing. We are often asked why we didn't. My stock answer is that the physicians did not ask me if they could practice medicine. Why should I ask them if I can practice nursing? My experience over the years in dealing with physicians is to take care to meet them on a one to one or small group basis, never en masse. As with all situations, questions and statements can be phrased in such a way that a "no" answer is unlikely. . . .

Mrs. W. is 72 years old and widowed. Her blood pressure was moderately elevated at first visit; she was obese and moderately tense. She had no physician and had had no physical examination for at least 5 years. We discussed the advisability of having a regular physician, especially since there might be need for evaluation of blood pressure readings such as those she had on her first visit. She expressed doubt about her ability to afford medical care, and we agreed that it might be possible to lower the readings if she would lose weight and learn to relax. Over the next 3 months she lost 7.5 pounds, but her blood pressure remained elevated (we use the Heart Association cutoff point of 140/90). Each time she came in for recheck of her blood pressure and general counseling I asked her if she had located a physician she felt she could trust and whom she could afford to see. Each time she said "No." I explained my misgivings about continuing to attempt to reduce her recalcitrant blood pressure without further diagnostic studies and probably medication—neither of which we could provide her. Finally I said that I was very uncomfortable seeing her continue to go without medical care. She suggested gently that she still was not convinced of the need to spend the money for something she did not think that important, and then she asked, "Does that mean you won't see me anymore unless I go to a doctor?" With that I realized that I had pushed her very close to feeling that she would be cut off from our services unless she did what we thought she should. I reassured her that my discomfort had nothing to do with seeing her and that we would continue to be available to her for whatever benefit she found in seeing us. She continues to come in more or less regularly; her blood pressure remains elevated, but she is learning to relax through experiments with yoga and meditation to which we referred her. In this instance we have had to deal with our feelings and concerns and really come to grips with the major premise we say we are there for—to help clients make informed decisions. The decisions are theirs, not ours, to make. . . .

Primary Care

Well-baby checks are made initially at 1 month by the physician. Subsequent visits are alternated between the physician and nurse practitioners. . . .

CPEs may be referred by a physician or by our central appointments referral system. . . .

Denver Developmental Screening Tests and Denver Articulation Tests are referred to me by a physician. . . .

Feingold diet consultations are referred by physicians to me. . . .

Rechecks, eg, otitis media, serous otitis, pneumonia, bronchitis, URI, diet follow-ups, etc, are referred by me, the physician, or central appointments. . . .

Crisis Care

Josephine Vander Meer, a specialized independent nurse practitioner in a family practice clinic, described one area of human crisis that makes up her practice. There is a large element of advocacy in this kind of practice.

Jo Vander Meer has worked for 2 years as an independent nurse practitioner on an interdisciplinary team in one program of the Family Practice Clinic of the Department of Family and Community Medicine at the University of New Mexico College of Medicine in Albuquerque. She has worked with sex offenders, with families of sex offenders, and with victims of sex crimes and their families. This is one of the few programs in the country that offers treatment to sex offenders and their families, as well as to victims and victims' families. At the time the Family Practice Clinic moved into this sex counseling program there was a 3-year history of an active rape crisis program in Albuquerque carried out by a group called the Task Force for Treatment of Victims of Sex Crimes. This group included members of many disciplines, including the police. It did a great deal to arouse community concern and to influence the care of victims of sex crimes. This group actively confronted the police and hospital personnel with the blaming, hostile, inhuman way this group of people were treated.

Jo, as a member of a team of four primary care providers, received clients through the emergency service of the County–Medical Center Hospital, where 90 percent of the victims of sex crimes are seen, although some were referred by police. Occasionally social workers, other hospitals, or the victims themselves refer to this team. Jo usually meets the victim of rape in the emergency room immediately after the occurrence of rape.

Incest victims most frequently come as referrals from the police. Incest victims are not usually identified as sex victims immediately. It may take a year or longer before the situation becomes known. Frequently some other crisis situation gets the problem out in the open. Sometimes it is the mother in the family who, while denying it, has been aware of the fact for a long time. When all her denial mechanisms fail she may report it; but this is rare. In Jo's experience she sees the mother, very often, as an active participant in this family dynamic. In one case the parents went to another state for the weekend. The daughter, feeling rejected by her stepfather because he chose the mother as a companion, told her girl friend. The friend's father just happened to be a policeman. When the girl friend told her father, it all came out. In another situation the event that precipitated the disclosure was that the incestuous father restricted the girl and would not let her have any social life. She, being unable to tolerate this, told her story. In another family, three stepchildren were all being sexually abused for a year and a half. The youngest child ran off with a girl friend and confided in her. The friend said that this had happened to her, too, that she had a stepfather who was molesting her. They went together to a neighbor's house and told their stories. The neighbor then called the police. The length of time between the onset of the incestuous relationship and the discovery by persons who can and will intervene often determines how much guilt the victims have mobilized by the time they get into treatment and accounts for the fact that the therapist may have to initiate contact with the client early in the treatment.

The sex offender almost always is referred to Jo or to members of her team by the police. These clients are in great contrast to the general population needing health care. Both offender and victim may deny that there is any problem, may deny the need for counseling, and may resist involvement in any kind of care system. Victims often feel shame and humiliation. Cultural values related to women who are raped tend to make them try to hide the fact that they have been raped. They are reticent to talk about what has happened to them. Offenders usually enter treatment in the hope of avoiding imprisonment or getting more favorable consideration from the court. These special problems of both victims and offenders require that the primary caretaker make the initial approach, and often succeeding approaches, in the greater number of cases.

Jo, a counselor, a physician medical faculty member, and an assistant physician comprise the primary care team; they take turns so that there is someone on call 24 hours per day, 7 days per week. Some member of the team sees every rape victim and incest victim, provides psychotherapy as needed, and helps the victim come to grips with the crisis in her life. Team members often help mothers, fathers, other family members, and boyfriends cope with their feelings so that they can be supportive with the victim. The team member who has the initial contact follows the client until discharge.

Jo's experience is that someone usually accompanies the victim to the hospital, especially if she is an adolescent. In early rape crisis work all the support went to the victim; but the family or boyfriend often experience such anxiety or rage that they also need help and often need medication. Frequently they need to come back to the clinic for help. She has also found that at the point of crisis the significant others are usually open and want to talk about the rape. If there are other siblings, parents often ask, "What do we say to the children?" With this kind of initial contact Jo has moved into their homes easily. Often they welcome her. She has also found that if she does not make a move in the emergency room or by telephone (or both), families tend not to use her at all. "It is not an easy subject to discuss. The victim has so much guilt placed there by society, and parents feel very guilty too." Depth in clinical skill is necessary in order to work with people who are not crying out for help, as well as to work with these families in their own homes in situations so much more complicated than the usual run of sexual problems. Jo sees the visits to the Family Practice Clinic as an avenue for these people to become involved in the health care system in new ways. Clients have said they didn't even know such a clinic was available and have begun to use it for other health problems.

Jo is convinced that a family approach to treatment of both offender and victim is the most useful. In incest the victim is playing one role, but the mother and father are playing complementary roles. In rape one often sees a family with an emotionally detached or absent father, as well as family disorganization and many other problems.

It is interesting that although the incidence of sexual abuse of children is supposed to be much higher than physical abuse, all the grants are being written and approved for physical abuse. People have a difficult time conceptualizing and talking about sexual abuse of children without becoming anxious—even professional people.

Nurses who work with victims of sex crimes and their families or sex offenders and their families need to consider carefully the issue of whose agent they are. Are they agents of the victim? The family? The victim's lawyer? The police? Legally, one has to say, "It depends." In some states nurse–patient communication is not privileged. Since being called on to be a witness in a court case is a good possibility, the nurse should know whether interview data are privileged before conducting an interview. Even if the data are privileged, it is almost impossible to represent someone or be an agent for someone at all times and in all situations. When the victim is underage, the contract for care is with the parent or, as in the case of incest, with the court or department of public welfare. The nurse must have a clear understanding of their expectations in terms of providing data about the client's sex life, her prerape behavior, or the events of the rape incident. It is very difficult after law enforcement officials have made a referral to refuse to assist in detection of crimes if the limits have not been set in advance. And police can exert a lot of pressure if mutually acceptable procedure is not agreed on in advance. The nurse also needs to have a clear understanding with the client before she provides the client's lawyer with information. She should know the rules of evidence and be familiar with methods of legal examination and cross-examination, since she will surely find her way to the witness stand as either therapist or expert witness or both.

Illness

I helped give a tub bath, counsel, and direction to a 75-year-old retired schoolteacher who lived with her son and daughter-in-law and their three girls. Care was indicated as this matriarchal former principal/teacher found it impossible to submit to family care in spite of her diabetes and Parkinson's disabilities. After bathing and personal care once weekly, we were all able to sit and casually discuss problems and solutions to them over a cup of coffee. On the evening of her death from a sudden coronary, the family called at 11 P.M. for counsel. I responded with a home visit (just minutes away), called a priest, and called a physician with a report of imminent death. I invited the family to have a rescue squad rush her to the emergency room; they declined and opted to notify the coroner and a mortician. This 2-hour visit satisfied the nursing needs of the intact family. . . .

A terminally ill patient discharged from the hospital 10 days previously after 2 months and $20,000 of hospital care had no local physician or referral for nursing care. His wife called me after seeing my name in the Yellow Pages. A physician was 50 miles away. After I made 19 daily visits giving enemas, medications, demonstrations, and support to the wife, a local physician saw him 5 hours prior to death to obviate (advocacy) the need for an out-of-county coroner and other problems that would burden the family further. The entire family was at his bedside at death. I consoled them. . . .

In psychiatric–mental health nursing the nurse needs to be able to take an extensive history and make a differential diagnosis. The nurse needs to know medical physiology. A 22-year-old college student came to me for sexual dysfunction therapy after being nonorgasmic for 1 year. She had been orgasmic previous to that. She responded to the workup with symptoms that sounded like diabetes to me. I referred her for a physical, and she was diabetic. She had a strong family history of depression and manic–depressive illness. I referred her to a psychiatrist, and she responded dramatically to antidepressant medication. She had not had a thorough workup in her previous therapy, and no history was taken. It was assumed by the therapist that her problems were environmental. . . .

With the higher risk factors in mind, we have tried to make special efforts to invite black clients in the pharmacy to talk with us and have their blood pressure checked. J.W., a 61-year-old taxi driver, noticeably overweight and wheezing with his chronic asthma, was in to buy a newspaper when I invited him to sit down. He told me he was under treatment at a nearby university and had been seen 6 months earlier. The blood pressure in his left arm was 210/120 and in his right 100/116. He knew this was much higher than it had been or should be; in fact, this was the highest he'd ever known it to be, but, "Usually they don't tell you what it is." He accepted my explanation of the severity of the reading and said he would act on the referral to return to the clinic as soon as possible. My telephone call 3 days later revealed that he had an appointment the following day. The next time our paths crossed in the pharmacy, he made a point of telling me that he had been admitted to the hospital when he went to clinic with both his blood pressure and his diabetes out of control. He said, "I probably wouldn't have made it if I hadn't gone when you told me to. You saved my life!" A bit of an exaggeration, but that's the kind of thing that makes it all worthwhile. . . .

Large numbers of critical incidents might reveal both the scope and frequency of various nursing practices. Structured critical incidents might have produced more comparable data than the free-form procedure used for the conference. In-depth nursing studies should ultimately permit definitive statements about the nature, usefulness, and value of nursing.

REFERENCES

1. Runyon JW, Jr: The Memphis chronic disease program. Comparisons in outcome and the nurse's extended role. JAMA 264:264, January 20, 1975
2. Chappel JA, Drogos PA: Evaluation of infant health care by a nurse practitioner. Pediatrics 49:871, 1972
3. Miller LV, Goldstein J: More efficient care of diabetic patients in a county-hospital setting. N Engl J Med 286:1388, 1972
4. Bessman AN: Comparison of medical care in nurse clinician and physician clinics in medical school affiliated hospitals. J Chronic Dis 27:115, 1974
5. Lewis CE, Resnick BA: Nurse clinics and progressive ambulatory care. N Engl J Med 277:1236, 1967
6. Miller LV, Goldstein J: More efficient care of diabetic patients in a county hospital setting. N Engl J Med 286:1388, 1972
7. Spector R, McGrath P, Alpert J, Cohen P, Aikens H: Medical care by nurses in an internal medicine clinic. Analysis of quality and its costs. JAMA 233:1234, 1975
8. Selected Bibliography with Abstracts in Joint Practice. Chicago, National Joint Practice Commission, 1975
9. Nader R: The $8 Billion Hospital Bed Overrun. Washington DC, 2000 P St, Health Research Group, 1975
10. Nurse Training, Health Revenue Sharing, and Health Services Act of 1976 (S66)
11. Kissam PC: Physician's assistant and nurse practitioner laws. Kansas Law Review 24:1, Fall 1975

CHAPTER 9

Nurse Practitioners and National Policy

One of the most encouraging signs in terms of national policy is the change in focus provided by the January 1975 National Health Planning and Development Act (PL 93-641). In essence, it says that up until this time every legislative act, whether for manpower training, program support, or provision of physical facilities, has been to produce more of the same. Now it is all to be changed. States will have to study their health needs, including manpower. All manpower is going to be looked at in terms of comprehensive health care. Nursing has an opportunity to define its service and delineate its contribution. But there are many problems to be solved.

ISSUES

Nursing leaders involved at the federal level in the development of national health policy are concerned about the nurse practitioner movement. They are concerned because they believe that many nurse practitioners are not addressing themselves to the health care problems of the nation. For example, while our greatest problem is maldistribution of health services, many nurse practitioners are not moving in to practice in underserved areas or to care for the poor wherever they are. Many nurse practitioners are addressing themselves and offering their services to the middle class, which the nursing leadership describes as already having adequate and effective care. There is concern because nurse practitioners are developing their practices around the fee-for-service concept and third-party payers. This appears to be a self-serving position at a time when on the national scene legislators are trying to do away with fee for service with its private incentive and the consequent maldistribution of health services. These leaders believe that nurses should talk about adequate reimbursement for services in terms of institutionalizing the fee-for-service model (agency-paid basis) to completely eliminate the profit aspect of practice. They claim fee for service can only further the present practice of nurse practitioners going into business where people can best afford to pay. One nurse sees a problem in the nurse practitioners' relationship to the system:

> Nurses are going out and setting up private practice because they've been trying to buck the system. They can't, and so they're going to do their own thing. I'm in complete sympathy with the people who have been trying to do it, because it's very hard to fight the system and achieve any input. I think I spend 99 percent of my time in this area. It is a difficult fight, but I think that nurses can get up and start putting in; trying to work with other people is hard work.

Some nursing leaders are concerned about criticism from the legislative branch of government for nurses' attempts to achieve fee for service. They are afraid that both lawmakers and the public will see nurses as just another special-interest group looking to rip off the people. There have been suggestions that nurse practitioners should underplay the fee-for-service concept and refrain from using private practice terminology, while talking more about what nurses have to offer as primary practitioners in health care services. These messages put nurse practitioners in conflict. These nurses, who are probably more active in politics and in the profession than the majority of nurses, see all of this toning down as a kind of doubletalk. If it is not interpreted as doubletalk, it is interpreted as urging the "mild, meek, good group of women" approach that nursing has used before. Such an approach can only benefit medicine and some of the emerging health disciplines that are competing with nursing for recognition, for status, and for money on the national level. The assumption that being devoted, good, and passive will ultimately win out has not proven true for nursing in the past. Nurse practitioners are put in a further quandary because many of them are extending and perpetuating the traditions of the medical model, which is and always has been supported by the private sector. One hears over and over questions that go something like this: "Can we in this country afford nursing growing up if this is what it means? Can't we bypass it? Do we have to go this route?"

MENTAL HEALTH AND COMPREHENSIVE HEALTH CARE

At the national health policy level there is interest not only in delivering health care to everyone but also in delivering comprehensive health care to everyone. The discipline of mental health–psychiatry has a 20-year history of support and practice outside of other health care settings. Much of the psychiatric nursing leadership is concerned first with existing legislation. The National Health Planning and Development Act, the precursor legislation to national health insurance, does not support the continued development of psychiatry in community mental health centers. If psychiatric services join with other health care services to the end of delivering comprehensive care, how will they move into the mainstream of health care? Second, there is concern that psychiatric–mental health nurse practitioners who are going into the private practice of nursing will have problems articulating their services with those of the nurse practitioners who offer primary care services and the programs of agencies developed for comprehensive health services. Leaders are concerned about further fragmentation of care, which is a major criticism of the existing health care delivery system. Some people think that nurses are rushing into private practice without having thought through their place in the system, or even what nursing approach they will follow. Heightened status and the possibility of higher income are seen as the major motivating factors for both independent and private practice. There is considerable concern that psychiatric nurses do not give total patient care. Counseling and psychotherapy are seen as inadequate in juxtaposition to total patient care. There is still concern that when a patient needs a bath, nurse practitioners teach the family how to do it, rather than doing it themselves. After 50 years of public health nursing, where family responsibility was always fostered, some nurses are still using this argument. Teaching, counseling, advising, advocacy, and support are not seen as "real" nursing by a group of nurses who believe that practitioners do these things because they are not committed to practice nursing. Some articulate nurses are critical of the number of nurse practitioners who specialize, saying that if national health policy develops in terms of primary and secondary health care, the majority of nurse practitioners will need to be primary care givers. Using the psychiatric–mental health nurse practitioners as an example, the rate at which they are going into private and independent practice would make for too large a group of nurses in secondary care. Other nurses who work at the policy level refuse to worry about this. They assume that it takes more than one group to do primary care, and they see psychiatric–mental health nurse practitioners as having significant functions in both primary and secondary care. Fragmentation worries seem groundless to them.

How nurse practitioners will use their power is of concern to some people. They are afraid that nurses will use their power to move the discipline ahead in terms of prestige and national influence rather than moving ahead in terms of health care delivery and innovative models for delivery of health care. They fear that nursing may be more interested in its own benefit than in the public need.

STANDARDS OF PRACTICE

Another policy issue is whether the majority of nurse practitioners are in fact expert practitioners. Nursing may have some grim realities to face in terms of getting at what is practiced, what kind of education is required for practice, and how to develop public confidence in nursing practice. One ultimate reality may be getting malpractice insurance. Certification by the American Nurses Association is one kind of assurance of knowledge about nursing care and medical practice, but many nurses think that certification is premature in terms of the state of nursing's body of knowledge. In any case, it is not mandatory for practice. One of the most frequently expressed needs of nurse practitioners is for ongoing or continuing education. This is often not available for community-based primary care or advanced therapeutic care. Peer review shows promise, but it is not operational in most settings where nurse practitioners work, for a variety of reasons. Some states, some insurance companies, and CHAMPUS (the coverage for military dependents) will pay nurses with master's degrees in their specialties. This is probably how government programs will be developed, ie, stating minimum qualifications for nurse practitioners. But if, as some nurses predict, all reimbursement is going to be completely medically controlled, nursing expertise will be determined by physicians.

STANDARDS OF PRACTICE AND REIMBURSEMENT

The federal programs may identify educational standards or specify supervision as a condition for reimbursement for services by nurse practitioners. This will in effect define one aspect of expertise (and possibly one safeguard) of the nurse practitioner's work. A variety of payers are waiting to see what the Social Security Administration turns up in terms of utilization of physicians' extenders. In a quasi-experimental study sponsored by that administration, a variety of practices are being selected for study.* The study will probably lean heavily on practice developed in the private sector. This quasi-experimental approach will reimburse services provided clients. Different levels of personnel will be paid at varying rates, with physicians receiving the highest rates. Some workers who are not in the usual health care system will not be reimbursed. The study will focus on utilization of providers on the basis of reimbursement. It will attempt to determine what happens to the practice economically, what happens when changes are made, what the patterns of practice are, and so forth. The study is in progress, but the reimbursement component is not expected to start until next year. Eventually Medicare and Medicaid will have policies concerning who is to be paid, for what, and at what rate.

Many nurse practitioners think that this study is too late and is not relevant to the problem. The federal government has supported training for many different kinds of health providers. This support has been given without collecting data on effectiveness and without performance data. This support has gone on for years, but now, after there are thousands of practitioners working whose training has been supported by the government, the government wants data before paying for their services. Everything is being held up for 1 to 2

**Robert Mendenhall, M.D., Medical Activities Manpower Staff, Dept. of Research and Medical Education, University of Southern California, School of Medicine, Rm 225 Keith Administration Bldg., 2022 Zonal Avenue, Los Angeles, California 90033, is conducting this project.*

years because the system of reimbursement is such that it does not provide for their being paid. Nurse practitioners are asking, "Why have we got this holding pattern?" Worse than that, even when the study is completed only a small part of the problem will have been addressed. Most of the practices studied are in the private sector; so in terms of fee for service there may be some answers. But in terms of fair salaries as reimbursement for skilled services, the study will not provide answers.

DEPENDENT, INDEPENDENT, AND INTERDEPENDENT NURSING PRACTICE

An important matter of policy at local, state, and national levels is whether the nurse may practice independently. If a nurse is permitted to carry her own primary care case load or patient group for treatment, while consulting with other professionals, collaborating with other professionals, and referring to other professions, that is one thing. But it appears in many practice acts that a great deal of nurses' duties are performed under the supervision of a physician. How this policy question is resolved in federal legislation and in nursing practice acts should make a vast difference in whether nurses practice mini-medicine, whether they deliver health care, or whether they do both. Or are nurses going to say that it does not matter what it is called or whether nurses have freedom to work with their own case loads? Nurses could say, "Only the care that people need is important. This is the only guideline we will use in policy development." If the greater part of a nurse's work is performing medical acts under supervision, and the remainder involves mother surrogate acts, there is little need for nursing licensure. The nurse operates on the physician's license in the first instance, and most women and many men can function as mother surrogates without a license.

The situation this nurse describes is not atypical as far as medicine–nursing relationships go:

I'm studying with a group of nurse practitioners, all of whom are graduates of our training program. As the training program has developed there have been a lot of maneuvers at the state level to set up constraints. We participate to develop practice content that deals with these constraints. One of the constraints is that of being appropriately tied in with physician backup. That's a reality. Essentially what I'm talking about is a formalization of the medical–nursing collaborative arrangements. It goes something like this: In order to practice as a nurse practitioner in this state, you have to be approved by a joint committee of the board of nursing and the board of medicine. The nature of this collaboration has to be approved. In order to practice, every nurse has to have at least successfully completed some training program or be certified by a training program. She also has to have a physician who is willing to work with her. There are problems with this interpretation, but in point of fact she is either employed by a physician, which some people worry about, or she is employed in a situation in which physicians are also employed and where there is at least one person who is willing to be her medical backup. There may be others. There has to be this kind of arrangement. We are finding out that the nurse practitioners are happiest when they have this kind of backup. They need it, and they do much better with a patient when they have it. The problems come when a client comes in and they have to refer this person to someone else at a later time because they do not know what to do. In other words, they can do their jobs as nurse practitioners when they have someone they can connect with. Their scope of practice is broad. The data we have suggest that nurses may overinvolve other people rather than underinvolve. In looking at analyses that have been done, you can be pretty certain that nurses are probably more cautious than incautious.

NURSING INPUT AT POLICY LEVEL

Nurse practitioners also need to guard against perpetuating the present system, and this can be done only at the policy level. What has happened (and it is common practice) is that physicians employ nurse practitioners because of the economic value of those services to them. Physicians, while not willing to allow nurses to practice privately, are willing to employ someone for whose services they can be reimbursed by all third-party payers. The economic value of a nurse practitioner's work can far outweigh the salary provided. Then the issues of distribution of care and comprehensiveness of care, which the nurse practitioner movement is all about, are overshadowed by concern for the economic value to the physician and economic exploitation of the nurse.

At the level of policy, nurses are concerned that they will not have opportunities under existing and proposed legislation to develop innovative health care delivery models. Nurses recognize that the medical model has become entrenched in its control of the way things get done and the manner in which problems are treated. Nurses would like to see collaborative, cooperative possibilities for care built into their health care models. They would like to try a system with an almost collegial decision-making network built into the system. They might have many kinds of backup from others in the system, so that the client would have multiple resources and would get into the kind of health-promoting situation he needs sooner than he would seeing one person in an office setting time after time. The concept of a single care provider is a kind of fragmentation in itself. Nurses want input in economic policy. As one nurse reports:

> We have a lot of specialists up on top who deal with the small part of the person, and the whole person never really gets taken care of. But if you have a primary care worker who can call on all of these specialists as needed, this can really bring the care right back to the family. They are doing it now at extremely high cost. Why should a physician's education be half-paid with tax dollars for 12 years or more of expensive training when people with just a few years of less expensive training can do as well as he can? Nurses who are practitioners are doing almost the same thing, with less training at less cost. I get a little uncomfortable when I see the nurse practitioner doing this kind of thing as well as a lot of physicians, but doing it at a fraction of the cost, in terms of the funds being spent on the training of each. The nurse practitioner movement is a windfall for the highly paid physician with nurses doing the work for little pay. If nurses had a systemic approach to the problem of health care delivery, it would bolster the position of nurses and help develop mechanisms to deal with the expenses of medical training.

Nurse practitioners want to be given public support and a high priority as they move into more responsible roles and into health-promotion work with clients. They recognize the public's commitment to medicine and the physician. They recognize the reality of the grasping medical system. They also recognize that they cannot effect change alone and that time and a variety of approaches to public support will be required for full public acceptance of nurse practitioners. But federal policy support is also important, and the National Health Planning and Development Act (PL 93-641) lists as its fourth national health priority "the training and increased utilization of physician assistants, especially nurse clinicians."

Nurses need to be involved in the policy issue of manpower distribution. No successful means have been developed to put health care workers where they are needed. Assistant physicians work a few years in a rural area and then move to the city where the lucrative practices are. Pediatric nurse practitioners did not stay in rural areas, but moved back to big cities to work in clinics and doctors' offices. Training indigenous health workers for underserved areas created multiple problems of acceptance by the group to be served and problems of referral to the few professionals. No one has found a way to pick up health professionals and to put them down where they are needed. Proposed federal legislation would tie federal support for education of physicians to a formal commitment to practice in underserved areas. This is another kind of trial, and nurses might take a position on this.

If nursing should want to tie nurse practitioner acceptance to improved health care, one nurse proposes this possibility:

> A very interesting approach that can be used is to look carefully at the population we begin with. We could take a lesson here from psychiatric social workers. They wanted to become independent practitioners. They went into the back wards that nobody wanted to be bothered with. Nobody wanted to compete with them there. And they began doing therapy. What happened before anyone knew it was that they had pretty well gotten themselves going and were a forceful group. If nursing is really concerned with delivering care to populations that don't have it, then it seems possible that we would get less flak than if we began to deal with the total population.

Support at the policy level for these kinds of activities might not only provide care but also permit the building of innovative health care delivery models.

Another idea that might be built into national policy relates to educational programs for nursing:

> I think you can place nurses strategically where they can help the cause of better care. You can't pick them up and put them down, but you can structure accessibility to certain things like educational programs. If you really want to change health care delivery, you do not set up a program in an institution and let anybody in. You think about where people come from and the potential of their remaining there. You build educational programs and make them available to these people, and you bring progress to them. We've done this in our state.

Educational programs routinely supported as a matter of public policy may be totally ineffective unless there is consideration of the system in which the graduate of the program is to work. Reimbursement for nurse practitioners in nursing homes is completely bottlenecked right now. The Department of Health, Education, and Welfare recently awarded seven or eight contracts to train geriatric nurse practitioners. This would meet a real need because of the terrible conditions of care in most nursing homes. But after these people are trained there will be no system for reimbursement. They cannot practice unless they occupy at least head nurse positions. So they add their geriatric nurse practitioner functions to other commitments and responsibilities. We are just not able to deinstitutionalize functions that have been institutionalized for so long, even though the function is not effective. What can nurses do in the face of this bottleneck in policy? What kind of positive input can they have? Some nurses want this kind of policy development:

> I think the solution has got to be on the national level, with financing mechanisms and reorganization mechanisms that will funnel dollars and resources into underserviced communities to reward all groups that provide needed services the same way.

Other nurses answer:

> Theoretically we agree with your strategy, but our understanding of the data that have come out on physician's assistants is that they initially start off in the rural areas, which presumably was the reason they were trained in the first place, but after 2 years of experience they end up in the cities.

It behooves nurse practitioners to support policy that puts all nursing practice within the mainstream of comprehensive health care. Legislation will probably be needed for this system-wide change, whether community mental health centers become comprehensive health care centers or whether other kinds of delivery systems find ways to articulate or plug into existing community mental health programs. Possibly both kinds of agencies and both kinds of programs will have to be modified before they can offer clients comprehensive care. Existing legislation does not appear to address this very real health care delivery problem. It is hoped that changes can be made that will eliminate the competition between the two models, much as elementary education is in a noncompetitive realm. The capitalistic model that medicine and the hospital bureaucracy have developed has fostered competition, and this will be difficult to resolve with or without a national policy on the problem.

SUMMARY

Nurse practitioners are interested in policies related to the health care delivery system and innovative health care delivery models. They are interested in policy that puts the consumer in the forefront and increases his options. They are interested in opening up the system so that consumers and care providers have the freedom to deal person-to-person rather than on a hierarchical basis. They are interested in motivating the poor to seek better health care. They are interested in focusing on health rather than illness. They are interested in a policy that will leave them free to utilize their skills fully and contribute to health care in real collaboration with other professionals.

Nurses who study various aspects of the health care system ask questions like these:

Where are we going with the nurse practitioner group, particularly because of the new legislation that allows practitioner capability that we haven't had before? What policies will develop related to this?

What contributions can research activity make to policy development? How can data be used by policymakers? What can researchers working with nurse practitioners do to raise questions that policymakers need to be thinking about? How can researchers working with nurse practitioners raise questions that generate more dynamic projects related to nursing? Should research activity be related to meaningful policy issues?

What effect do nurse practitioners have on other kinds of nursing personnel? What effect are nurse practitioners having on the major problems of health services delivery?

There are more nurses studying federal and state policy than ever before. It is an interesting and critical area right now:

> The fact that nurses have moved so far in 4 or 6 years is absolutely astounding. When the idea of primary care nursing was presented at a meeting 6 years ago, people said, "Isn't it interesting? But where would these people work?" We have come a long way. There is no area in this country that doesn't know about primary care nursing. We have many

groups that are deeply involved. This is exciting. Nurses are really involved.

But amid the excitement one nurse adds a note of caution:

It is important that policy be made with knowledge of all the facts and with a broad look at all the different kinds of models. Before making policy about practitioners, we must make sure that there has been adequate thought input; because once the policy has been made, we're stuck with it.

CHAPTER 10

Research Issues

When independent and private practitioners of nursing think about research, they must first ask, "What questions are really important for us to address?" The answer to this question should determine the selection of what will be researched. With each innovation in the nursing profession there have been pleas for research prior to implementation; the pleas go something like this:

> I would love to see a first in nursing history. It may already be too late, but I would like to see us get ourselves together before we go off on the practitioner tangent. Nursing has run off half-cocked on every little and big thing that has come along, time and time again. I think it has been to our detriment, and I think, for once, we should get ourselves together before we pursue this new route for nursing. It would be a blessing.

The need for careful research designed to answer relevant questions is paramount for the nurse practitioner movement. Not only will the questions determine the research to be done, but the answers will influence how research will be used in introducing innovations and in the whole process of change. The issue is not just doing research. If nurses do research that does not relate to the concerns of the public, its usefulness may be limited and its value lost, at least for a period of time.

POLITICAL USE OF RESEARCH FINDINGS

The usual assumption is that research involves a search for scientific truth, and this should, of course, be true of research done about the nursing practice of nurse practitioners. The findings of such research should be used in the customary ways, but nurses are beginning to be aware that research findings can also be powerful political tools that can be used both for and against their interests. This recognition is particularly important today if nursing is to stand with other professions, compete with them in the arena in which health care decisions are made, expand the scope of reimbursable health care services, and receive adequate reimbursement for the nursing component of these services.

In addition to the problem of formulating relevant research questions about nursing, there is the problem of how to get the research findings heard once they are completed. The other health care professions, as well as the public, often have not been willing to listen to and accept the results of research that contradicts traditional belief or practice. This is not unique to nursing, but it may be a crucial problem for nursing today. As we have already been reminded by the studies of nurse midwives at the Frontier Nursing Service in Hyden, Kentucky, in spite of demonstrations that the use of nurse midwives can significantly reduce infant and maternal mortality and morbidity, most states will not permit them to practice, even within carefully defined limits. They would constitute an economic threat to physicians.

During the past few years a number of studies of nurse practitioner practice have been done, and the results have been disseminated among health professionals. For example, Dr. Reynold Spector and associates at the Peter Bent Brigham Hospital Internal Medical Clinic in Boston did a 3-month study of five selected nurses caring for 174 patients who were referred by 78 of the 115 physicians staffing the clinic in a total of 403 visits.[1] Nurses were judged in a variety of ways. Ninety-eight percent of the time the nurses carried out physicians' orders correctly. They identified 107 new health problems, but according to the strict medical criteria used for analysis, they handled only 85 percent of them correctly. Scheduled visits to the physicians and unscheduled visits to the emergency room decreased, but visits to the nurses increased. The overall cost of care for the study patients increased 24 percent during the 3-month period, and patient care was not judged to be improved. The sample was small, the 3-month training of the nurses was not specified, and the patient referrals were not all common medical problems. Many had psychiatric or social problems, and many were referred for medication check (whatever that means). Also, how the nurses were supported while moving into the new roles was not specified, nor is mention made of whether 3 months is enough time to develop comfort in the roles, even though the nurses had been in the clinic for a year.

Often, incomplete short-term projects that are not well planned or controlled are carried out. The results of these studies are then published in prestigious journals and treated as if they were as valid as carefully controlled experimental studies. Thus used, they provide support for maintaining the status quo in health care delivery. Certainly the contribution of nursing to health care delivery should be studied carefully, but the quality of the research should be considered before it is used to support any position.

The character of the public and professional mix is changing every year. The public is becoming stronger and demanding more input in health care planning and in maintenance of high-quality care. A case in point is the Professional Standards Review Organization (PSRO). The medical profession did not ask for it and certainly is not happy with it, but it is a reality. This call for accountability took precedence over the resistance put up by the medical profession. It is important to note, because it is a beginning. We are moving into a period where, if we have good data to present, the public will listen. At least we need to put our research house in order so that we can capitalize on opportunities for nursing when they come.

STUDYING NURSING: THE ISSUES

There are several camps in the nurse practitioner movement. There is agreement on some issues among some camps, but there are also major differences. One group is looking toward redefining nursing without giving up traditional functions and without taking up the slack caused by medicine's shortcomings. This group fears that some other group will emerge and take over nursing's traditional functions, leaving nursing with nothing but medical functions under the supervision of physicians. This group is concerned that those who practice medicine under medical supervision will insist that they are practicing nursing and will not be honest enough to admit that they are extenders of the physician, nor admit that they are technical workers, not professional workers. In terms of its theoretical frame of reference, this group rejects a disease orientation for nursing, even when it comes to disease prevention as contrasted to health achievement, health maintenance, and health promotion. Adherents to this position believe we must define nursing and must start with the client to do it. They maintain that we have never asked the client what his needs are and what he wants of us. They insist there must be a body of knowledge for nursing that is not just medical.

Another group believes that it is difficult if not impossible to identify what nurses do as distinguished from the work of the other members of the team, to tease out nursing's contribution when everyone is working on the patient at once. They believe that only the patient can define nursing, but the patient is often limited to relating his emotional reaction, since he usually does not have the scientific knowledge and conceptual skill to define his view of nursing succinctly. This group asks, "Do we really care what the nurse does, or what is important in terms of determinants?" They are interested in what works and why, and they do not ask questions about who does what. They think doctors may make good or poor nurses and that nurses may make good or poor doctors, but what is relevant is the effectiveness of health care. When asked about a health focus, they say the question of health always leads to the question of what is normal. Three-quarters of the population each month report one or more problems that are medical in nature. There are very few people who are completely free of some symptom or health problem, and the general expectation is that there will never be a population free of these kinds of problems. The health care delivery system right now is functioning on the medical model. Should not nurses face reality? This reality is that medicine is in charge. Nursing needs to learn medicine and do primary care because society needs primary care. Nursing needs to ask these questions: What kind of contribution can nurses make in the existing system? What is the effectiveness of nursing practice in the health care delivery system? Another reality is that we are dealing with a society that enters the health care system with a complaint of some sort. Maybe the client has to label it illness or make up an illness label to get into the health care system, and maybe we should study that.

A third group of nurses is similar to the second group in subscribing to the team approach and believing that overlapping of functions should not be of concern. They argue strongly for nurses developing competence in the medical area, citing the advantage of greater integration in the delivery of care to patients. They resist getting bogged down in consideration of their relationships with medicine and whether they are helping medicine deliver medical care.

Nurses feel strongly about the positions they take. This fact and the fact that there is such great polarity among positions will not permit selection of only a single set of research questions for nursing. Each camp generates very different questions. But this may be a more effective approach than to predict needs and design nursing programs on the basis of statistics that originate with the pathology orientation of the medical profession, which is the approach that generally has been followed thus far in development of nurse practitioner programs and in studies conducted to evaluate their impact.

STUDYING NURSING: IS THERE A UNIQUE CONTRIBUTION?

Nurse practitioners must address the question of what they need to know about themselves. If they cannot answer this question, they cannot help anybody else understand their nursing services or the importance of the movement in health care delivery. The easier questions to research are those related to cost–benefit analysis and unit costs. It may be fairly easy to demonstrate that nurse practitioners reduce inpatient days. There has already been some research in this area.

The questions that are extremely difficult to formulate and answer are qualitative ones. It is often the quality of the experience that the client has with the nurse that makes the nursing care worth professional-level fees. Nurses are the professionals best prepared to promote physical, psychologic, and social benefits for living. Many nurse practitioners are relating to communities in terms of expressed needs and are working with the client rather than doing things for the client. They are taking roles as facilitators in problem-solving; they are getting and using information. More than merely fostering and supporting survival and coping, they improve the quality of life through promoting growth and learning. Such benefits are difficult to measure for research purposes, and they are difficult to explain to an audience. For example, it may be difficult to convince an audience of the value of changing the way people feel.

But social and psychologic benefits must be demonstrated if nurse practitioners are to receive recognition as health care providers and reimbursement for nursing services. It may not be enough to document benefit. Nursing also may have to convince other professionals, if not the public, of the relevance of social and psychologic benefits to the discipline of nursing. We need to be clear that the general focus of the past on "What do nurses do?" must now change so that the focus is on "What contribution does nursing make?" And in relation to the health care system, we may need to stay with the question, "What nursing is needed?" In any discussion of the question of whether nurses need to do more research on the process and effectiveness of health promotion, someone always raises the question of how health is defined and whether there is a need to study the ramifications of health and the public conception of it. One nurse spoke on this issue from her experience:

> Your definition of health reminds me of the little old lady I saw the other day. She is 86 years old. She'd had a CVA and walks with a limp. She can hardly eat anymore. She is blind in one eye. But she was very happy she was well again. She was not feeling sick; she felt she had been rehabilitated; she felt good.

For some nurses there is an interest in doing research that differentiates nurses from other health care workers. There has been concern about the need to compare differences in processes and outcomes between the physician's assistant and the clinical specialist, for example. Other researchers appear to be moving from that level of question to documenting the ways in which nursing functions are promoting health. But it is difficult in a profession so beset with identity problems to put away the question of how well nurses can perform functions in comparison to other health care workers. Janet Ruffin cites this example:

> In a multi-disciplinary setting which utilizes nurses in "expanded roles," I think there are problems with determining which research is most relevant. These nurses are raising questions about the boundaries of their roles: what is nursing, and what does a nurse do differently from a "generic mental health worker" of any given discipline or experience background; how can we evaluate the quality of their performance if all staff function with the same responsibilities for clinical care? Our concerns in the Department of Nursing are not the common ones of facilitating nurses' being allowed to function in autonomous ways. Instead, we are concerned that the nursing identity is being lost in

the context of a setting which identifies everyone as a generic mental health worker. Administratively, some questions are: whether to resist this erosion of nursing identity by devising research which "proves" that there are differences among staff in terms of task performance; or, to direct energies toward evaluation of quality of care without regard for the staff worker's identity.

Another nurse cites this example:

This is what the Burlington Study in Canada found in using nurses prepared as family nurse practitioners. The physicians think it is so successful; they talk about the successful demonstration of the nurse practitioner role. Well, it was successful because the nurses did about as well as the physicians did in prescription of drugs and management of the patients in the medical sense. Nurses' outcomes weren't any worse than the physicians. Therefore it was successful. Then you turn around to the nursing community and say it wasn't very good at all, and the reason was a very good one—that the patients served by the nurses didn't show any better progress than the patients served by the physicians. In a recent conference some nurses were critiquing this study and criticizing these people for the fact that they didn't study everything that was going on. The question for nurses belonging to this movement might be: What is the least possible amount of medicine that can be taught to do acceptable medical management? This is what this study apparently says—that the nurses who had considerably less medical education were getting outcomes that were no worse than those of the physicians. Therefore, you give nurses one-sixteenth of the training. That has marvelous implications. Why prepare these expensive physicians if you can get a quickie to do the same thing? But that does not mean they have good care.

This particular study has opened up new vistas to a lot of people.[2] It has had a policy impact. People are now going to have nurses participate in certain kinds of care because they can do it. However, the point is that it has not done a thing in terms of improving our understanding of how to manage patients, how to manage care, or how to make clinical decisions. Its impact is in opening up options that weren't there before. But the question is this: Will our practice and the research of our practice lead us to a position where we can contribute to the resolution of problems or the prevention of problems? Will we contribute something that makes sense in clinical management, as opposed to just determining whether we use this type of worker or that type of worker? There are two major problems. One concerns what kind of research we want to do and what kind of data we want to gather so that we can make the points we need to make in the public domain and in the political arena. The other problem concerns policy. How can we aid the people who are making policy, and how can we have a voice in making sure that policy is made on the basis of adequate hard data and accurate interpretation of data?

REFERENCES

1. Spector R, McGrath P, Alpert J, Cohen P, Aikens H: Medical care by nurses in an internal medicine clinic: analysis of quality and its costs. JAMA 233:1234, 1975
2. Spitzer WO, Sackett DC, Sibley JC, et al: The Burlington randomized trial of the nurse practitioner. N Engl J Med 290:251, 1974

CHAPTER 11

Other Issues

HEALTH VERSUS ILLNESS

Every month 75 percent of the population reports one or more illnesses or medical problems. Very few people are completely symptom-free. Regardless of how the symptoms are coded, as functional, malfunctional, or pathologic, this is a very high percentage of a supposedly healthy population to be having complaints. Medicine accepts these figures and projects that we will never have a population free of these kinds of problems. But one can also look at the situation from another point of view. Nurse practitioners recognize that health care delivery is still operating out of the medical model. It is still a medical care delivery system. "Something is wrong and we must cure it" has been the thought pattern in medicine for generations. Complaint is the language of illness, and it has been carried over to the more recent concern with health. Complaint is the accepted way to focus attention on one's health or one's functioning, and if one is to be admitted to the health care system one must have and be able to explicate a respectable symptom. People who rejoice in their health and exclaim about the joys of being alive may be thought to be a little odd or may be subject to ridicule, unless they use poetry. What short shrift one would get if apprehended trying to edge into the health care system by presenting the symptoms of one's growth and development or good health. One gets little enough recognition and only grudging admission for the six most common discomforts (nausea and vomiting, diarrhea, headache, sore feet, low back pain, and upper respiratory infection). For many workers in the health care system, health is conceptualized as disease prevention. While disease prevention may be the bridge between the disciplines of pathology and health, it has little to do with health promotion, health support, or other concepts of human existence.

A whole new body of knowledge about health has come into existence, but it is not operational in the lives of people except in minimal or fragmented ways. New structures need to be developed to deliver health care, and these structures must be linked with the existing medical care system. We need to develop a new language of health needs and integrate it not only with the language of health professionals but also with the vernacular. Nurse practitioners are in an ideal position to make a real contribution to the accomplishment of these tasks. Nursing was one of the first disciplines to be committed to patient teaching and health supervision. It already has a health orientation. It needs structures within which to develop health practices and to research health. Nurse practitioners, because of their own work and their observations of the way the medical care system operates, are in an excellent position to develop and test new structures for health care delivery. Nurses can develop structures and practices for maintaining, achieving, and promoting health that can turn this kind of practice around. For example:

> I saw a family where the combined years of psychotherapy were 76 years, and no one had ever identified the strengths in this family. They were initially told, and this was a professional family, "You are in bad shape. It will take years to get you better." It was appalling. They were really on their way to health when all we did was identify their strengths. In our agency we threw out the idea of "What is wrong with you?" and said, "For God's sake, look at the health strength that kept this gutsy family going all these years."

Another does it this way: "One of the basics I have developed in my family practice is that people can call me and say, 'Come to us in our own home where our real strengths are, and let us talk with you about this problem.' " It is probably impossible for people to get good health care out of the medical model of care delivery, no matter how health care is added to the disease model of medical care. If a mother takes her child to a pediatrician because she's concerned about something and the physician finds nothing wrong, he may well foster in her a sense of being wrong and by implication let her know that she has wasted his time. But if he has a health-supporting orientation he can tell her instead that she is a good mother, as well as help her to identify the ways in which she is doing a good job and assess with her the child's new growth and developing attributes. He might even project new developmental tasks, teach her how these occur, and outline the things that will facilitate full flowering of the abilities that accomplish these tasks.

Employees of the Frontier Nursing Service, which has provided health care for a certain rural population over several generations, think that they see positive results from the vast amounts of teaching done over the years. The people are much more knowledgeable about health. They find daughters and granddaughters who know what was taught to the first generation of mothers. Family members know more about promoting the health of the family and more about self-care. No formal studies have documented these changes. They also have no statistics to substantiate what they observe to be decreases in divorce rates, juvenile delinquency, and morbidity. There has been a great decrease in the use of hospital beds by members of the community over 65 years of age, with greater family responsibility for care at home. These are the kinds of studies nurses need to do.

The problem-solving skills needed in dealing with the evolving process of healthy living and the healthy life are not built in, and people bog down at times of change. Mothers have a hard time sending their children to school or letting them leave home to go to college; they have problems dealing with adolescent behavior. Couples get into hassles in planning their weddings. There are all kinds of people whose problem-solving skills are not adequate for handling the myriad stresses that occur in families, and these people have nowhere to get assistance unless they can be diagnosed as maladjusted, inadequate, or sick. The system is so strong and has so influenced cultural values that individuals and families feel guilty for breakdowns in problem-solving skills. It is interesting to note that they cannot be understood by use of crisis theory, partly because definitions of crisis are so pat and partly because to do so would identify them as sick. There is little room in crisis theory for minicrises in living or blocks in problem-solving. This becomes more obvious when one looks at treatment of people who are in crisis: there are few problem-solving activities, few educative activities, few health assessments, little consideration for growth-producing or maturing experiences, and little concern for building their strengths or for using the resources at hand (in self and family). The family is identified as being in crisis and is immobilized. Crisis theory has only recently taken into account that there are tremendous variations in responses to problems. What represents a crisis for one person or one family may be only an event in the lives of a hundred others. This reveals that there is a great deal of strength that people have ready to bring to bear in solving their problems.

MEDICAL MODEL VERSUS INNOVATIVE MODELS OF HEALTH CARE

The medical model has been and still is a closed model for an elite group of practitioners. The client may be referred and pushed from one component of the model to another, but he is kept within the model for all treatment. If ultimately he cannot utilize or respond to what the model has to offer, he is labeled recalcitrant, stubborn, intractable, chronic, or hopeless. Resources outside the model are not considered in terms of what they have to offer the client, either at the point of assessment or at the point of medical failure. A few nurse practitioner models are built on an open-system concept. Even with so-called comprehensive care no system is going to meet all the expressed needs of clients. These nurses respond to this by working out with the client what his needs are and how he conceptualizes solutions to his problems. In situations where the agency does not have the necessary resources, these nurses have built a large supporting structure of resource people in the community. Some of the resource people are professional, although such people as educators, members of the religious establishment, acupuncturists, chiropractors, bioenergetic specialists, artists, and musicians might not be considered as therapists with primary therapeutic responsibility in a medical care service. A large group of former clients and clients who have successfully dealt with particular types of crisis is also available. No effort is made to keep the client in the system or to force him to use only those resources within the system. Every effort is made to find the help that clients think will be comforting, supporting, enriching, face-saving, shame-minimizing, etc. One agency's policy is described this way:

There are so many options that you get attitude changes about being possessive. And I've seen the organization change. For example, a couple came to us about 2 months ago. Another staff member and I did a 2-hour evaluation. It's always a two-person evaluation. The husband and wife really wanted a physician. Regardless of what our input was, they wanted a medical opinion. The husband said, "My wife has a medical problem." The wife said, "The medical thing wrong with me is that they removed my breast—they did something to me." It was clear that no one on our staff could supply what they were asking for. Our physician is in general practice problems, and he was not going to say the things they wanted to hear. We laid it out for them: "We don't think we're the people who are going to help you." They said, "We'd like to try." They tried for 6 weeks, meeting with one of our therapists. It was disaster. We had already referred them to a large medical center in the metropolitan area and a good internist with whom they were delighted. It would have been a hassle to keep referring them within our organization, even though they were willing.

The medical model controls all the rewards. The old Hill-Burton legislation rewarded everybody for building hospitals, not health centers or preventoria. The National Health Planning and Development Act (PL 93-641) gives high priority and support to the further definition of illness and disease. Nurse practitioners, if given a small fraction of the support presently allocated to developing the medical model, could develop and test health-promotion models of care and could experiment with ways to articulate the two types of models—medical care and health care.

The medical model, even with some improvement in the last decade or so, is a paternalistic, essentially authoritarian model for the delivery of care. This model is much more apt to foster dependency than to produce growth and strength. It is much more likely to specify what the client's needs are at all levels than to listen to either a client's or a community's own identification of needs. This process of invalidation operates from the premise that the client is weak rather than strong. If a couple has been living together 20 years and then begins to wonder why, how could they be expected to get their dilemma solved in this kind of system? There must be a lot of strength there. There is a tendency among all middle-class professionals to focus on the weaknesses of the poor. Even there one must recognize the strength inherent in surviving in spite of poverty.

Consumers have picked up the challenge of health care. They are now spearheading the movement and are beginning to define what kind of health care they want. It appears that consumers are saying they want to be in charge of their health care. While illness care has top priority, health care is gaining ground. Consumers want to be listened to, and they want their concerns dealt with seriously. Many consumers want to have health care in their own homes, if possible. Consumers want to be considered as holding a position of strength. They want to know the options, they want to have input in setting up the options, and they want to choose the option they prefer for health care. Consumers no longer want professionals unilaterally defining their needs and identifying their options. The old paternalistic approach may be as bad as offering nothing at all. If we dictate what is good for people, we then use all our energies manipulating people toward that good.

Some nurses have accepted the theory that clients should choose their own experience or make their own experience and that it is unethical to tell a client that the experience he has chosen for himself is not good for him. The creation of life experiences is unique and quite remarkable. Health professionals may help identify options and may project risks and various types of outcomes, but the client chooses. There have been glaring examples of failure of the medical model, as in treatment of diabetes and cardiac patients or treatment of alcoholism and obesity. Some nurses are recognizing that the options we lay out for people are not really options in their frame of reference because of cultural, economic, or other differences that are not considered in identifying the options. Nurses are also beginning to look at new models, recognizing that most of what has been done in terms of a real health care program has been lip service, a game people have been playing since recognition of the vast neglected area of health promotion. One of the problems health maintenance organizations have had is that they have not sold health promotion or offered identifiable health promotion services. Instead, they have offered testing and screening, where a search for illness, not health, was the goal.

By the time of World War II health professionals rarely saw clients in their homes. Except for community health nurses, few health workers ever saw the patient's home. There were good reasons for this, in terms of cost of care and facilities for diagnosis and care in the home and in terms of the shortage of health care workers. Nurses are becoming aware that much information about symptoms, diagnosis, therapeutic regimens, and quality of life is lost if the client is not seen in his home. As one nurse noted, the client's medicine closet may be an arsenal of drugs that counteract or potentiate each other, or health practices may be at a minimum because of a variety of family dynamics. Also, nurse practitioners have found that a large percentage of their clients prefer to do most of their work with health care professionals in their homes. Insofar as is possible, nurses are building this into their practices, and corporations are providing for home care in their policies relating to care. Home care increases costs, but whether it reduces illness, decreases the use of hospital beds, makes people more effective in meeting their own health needs, or enriches their lives requires determination by research or at least some demonstration.

Some nurses contemplate a kind of free-floating model for health care delivery. This model would be constructed to respond to the expressed needs of the community as individuals seek assistance. This model would have to be developed in such a manner that it would be culturally acceptable to people seeking help. A few nurses who have gone into practice on the premise of being responsive to community needs have found themselves teaching clients how to assess their own state of health, how to assess the health of their children, how to keep from getting senile, and how to intervene in problems of privacy, personal space, grief, loss, and job dissatisfaction. They work at helping people face change and alter their life styles. They work at helping people find meaning. Essentially, they deal with all the health concerns that individuals and families have over the span of life. Clients want someone who can listen to them and offer them feedback to facilitate the use of their own resources.

Nurse practitioners can address themselves to relating to the normative mode in our society. A breakdown in normal daily activities of individuals or families may be the point at which nurse practitioners can make their best contribution, by being available to support the integration and growth of the individual or family. Nurse practitioners do have greater freedom to use alternatives for care than nurses who work within existing systems.

There is still considerable missionary spirit among nurses. There is concern for the poor and for improving their economic situation, as well as their nutrition, housing, and job stability; nurses are searching for ways to work with professionals outside the health system to resolve these problems. It is very difficult to be guided by what the poor say they need. It is much easier to decide what is good for the poor, what would make for a better life. In some ways nurses are hardly better prepared to deliver health care to the poor than physicians are. We must be careful; precisely because we are change agents we must be careful that we do not cut out a segment of the population and say what they really want. Even talking about motivating the poor implies known outcomes or goals. Support for health care from official agencies may not allow nurses to free-float in this area, since both goals and methods will be built into the legislation.

CONTROL OF PRACTICE VERSUS SUPERVISED PRACTICE

Must a profession control all aspects of its own practice and accredit or license those who practice? Can one be said to have a profession when some of one's functions partake of a second profession, when these functions are delegated as well as supervised by the second profession, and when the second profession insists on accrediting the members of the first profession who practice the delegated tasks? Nursing, of course, would like to be a profession and would like to control its own practice, regardless of answers to these questions.

It might appear that the efforts toward freedom in nursing, as well as changes in medical practice acts in 41 states and nursing practice acts in 28 states, have gained more authority and autonomy for nurses. In other words, the new laws could be expected to permit nurses greater freedom to practice in expanded roles and give them greater control of that practice. Actually, the changes in the medical practice acts authorize delegation of medical authority. So, as far as medicine is concerned, medicine still supervises and controls medical practice and delegated medical functions. For all practical purposes, medicine can be defined as all acts of patient care that physicians are trained to perform.[1]

Eighteen of the new nurse practitioner statutes require some form of regulation, administered most often by joint action of the medical and nursing licensing boards. Ten states' new statutes "authorize expanded medical delegation . . . without explicitly authorizing an administration agency or professional society to regulate the process."[1] Some states, even without a statute, are developing regulatory procedures, and it appears that these procedures authorize the nurse to perform any delegated act provided the supervising physician ascertains that she is qualified.[1] Hall notes that "the New York definition [of nursing practice] is much more sophisticated than the traditional definition. However, analysis of it reveals that it does not extend the scope of nursing practice in the medical area beyond the traditional concepts."[2] The California nursing practice act contains a preamble that recognizes nursing as a dynamic, evolving field with overlapping and mutually shared functions with medicine. The intent of the legislation is to give legal backing to those functions that become commonly used in nursing. This law may have possibilities in terms of nursing control of nursing practice if the definition of nursing is not interpreted too narrowly.

But the answers to whether the situation will change so that nursing can control its own practice are to be found in the realm of the politics of medical care delivery rather than in studying changes in the various state laws, and past experience tells us that change in terms of control of practice is unlikely. Medicine has consolidated its power to influence legislation effectively to eliminate economic threats and threats to its control. Organized medicine does not permit competition, and this lack of competition maintains physicians' fees at high levels. Physicians' fees have increased much faster than the overall consumer index.[1] If physicians will not allow competition among themselves without threat of expulsion from the medical society or revocation of license, it is a certainty that they will attempt to eliminate any threat posed by nurse practitioners. There is no question that at this time organized medicine at both the state and national levels has the power to do it.

Several nurses in the conference group have had pressure put on them. One well-trained and experienced nurse practitioner was told by a board of medical examiners that she could not call herself nurse practitioner, that she could use only the single word nurse. The secretary of the board of nursing told her to take it easy, that the situation was very delicate. Another nurse practitioner was told to close down her practice after a board of medical examiners went to the state attorney general and complained that she was practicing medicine. She closed her practice and told her clients the reason. The governor and the attorney general were inundated with complaints, and the practice was soon allowed to reopen. One well-known practitioner, one of the early pioneers, was accused by the physicians on the state joint practice committee of practicing medicine. She openly admitted that she was practicing medicine under the supervision of a physician and asked whether they shouldn't take up their complaint with the physician. A physician who was functioning as backup to a nurse withdrew with the explanation that he was up for his permanent license to practice in a few months and there had been hints that he might not get that license if he continued his support of the nurse practitioner. It has already been noted that one state board of medicine, without informing the board of nursing, made a surprise inspection visit to a nurse practitioner's office. There have been many other instances, but only one conferee was willing to have her name linked with the incident. So great is the fear of medical retribution!

While the pressure is on to provide good medical care to the minorities, the poor, the aged, and the rural population, physicians will work with nurses and others. With the assistant physician there is no question about delegation and supervision. Colleague relationships, joint practice, and collaboration in practice with nurses very often mean supervised practice in a sponsorship or employee–employer relationship. At the operational level many physician–nurse practitioner collaborative arrangements are exemplary. But at the policy level medicine dictates, at best, carefully controlled expansion of medical delegation.[1] Several nurses in the conference group even had problems with medicine related to charging fees as high as physicians' fees.

It may be best to be a satisfied, supervised nurse practitioner who does not threaten the physician sponsor or employer economically or in practice—at least for some period of time.

It may be that nurses should redirect their energies to develop the large gray areas of sociopsychiatric, educational, facilitative advocacy and health-promoting skills to add to their armamentarium of comfort skills so that they can control some of their practice.

It may be that nurse practitioners can control their practices in certain contexts. In one group there was some discussion about one of its nurse practitioner members who was doing extensive primary care and why the physicians had not challenged her. One nurse speculated:

> Do you think some of the reasons you don't get flak about overstepping is because you're in a position where a physician wouldn't desire to go, and if you moved into a high-class community, it would be potentially taking away from his clientele? He's not going to go out on the Indian reservation or Alaska or whatever, or into a lower-class population. He's more than content to have you fill those health needs. . . .

A related interchange went like this:

> PARTICIPANT: I'd say that better than half of the people we see would prefer to do most of the therapy within their homes. But one of the things that gets into is this question: Who pays for that kind of time, and who but nurses will go there?

PARTICIPANT: In a poor community, obviously economically that's not possible, but it's also not possible because the professionals aren't there. And they're not going to get there. You can wait 20 years and they still won't get there. . . .

Another nurse describes the flak she gets:

We can't get our clients to see a dentist because they cannot pay. A lot of these families are large families, and they can't afford dental care. It gets last priority. If there is any money left, it goes for anything but dental care. So the ones I'm getting flak from are the dentists, because we take care of those kids' dental problems, the adults' too, but primarily children. Our clinic doesn't offer dental health care, so I went to the Army Reserve, and they had dentist reservists who donated their time at the clinic. I am really getting it from the dentists. I also went to the doctors in the Army Reserve. We now have 16 doctors who come out to our clinic on Saturdays. That's the only time I had a doctor. I went to the National Guard and got their doctors for Thursday night, so I have a doctor there at least one night a week. I didn't get the same response from the civilian doctors. They think it's a neat idea that army doctors are coming out; but the dentists are furious! The dental association won't have any part of us in any way. I tried to go through them to get fluoride treatments and a preventive program for the kids. You know how dentists believe in prevention? They wouldn't listen to me. They wouldn't even let me talk to them. They are really against it, because they think I'm taking their money away from them. But they wouldn't get the money. I've seen 3-year-olds with just stubbles in their mouths where their teeth are already all gone. At 3 years old that's really bad. I thought I'd approach them from that angle. If I could get these guys to come out and do dental care on these kids and give them treatment and they saw these mouths, they wouldn't object to it. But I couldn't even get my foot in the door.

It may be that certification, especially if it retains its medical orientation, will provide more freedom for the nurse practitioner to control her practice. While it may be reasonable to hope for this, one cannot ignore the results of past struggles with the power structures.

An entirely different approach would be to ignore who delegates what and who supervises what and for a period of years put all of the profession's energies into providing, describing, and refining health care. Then, farther on down the road, we could define ourselves and lay claims to our territory. This would be a lovely plan if medicine and society retained the status quo, but effective health care policy is probably not going to wait.

INDEPENDENT VERSUS AGENCY PRACTICE

The private practice of nursing is about as emotional an issue for nurses as fee for service. There is less argument generated by joint practice, sponsored practice, or practice with a hospital or clinic. One could view the issue from a variety of points of view. Some nurses rejoice that nurses have a service to offer that will support a private practice. At some level nurses recognize private practice as one place the body of knowledge of nursing will continue to grow. There are those who believe it is long overdue that medicine be confronted with the limitations of the medical model for promoting health. And there are those who think it is time that medicine's power and omniscience be challenged. On the other hand, there are those who think that private practice bodes ill, that it is passé, that it fragments health care and confuses the public, and that its practitioners are prestige-driven and money-mad.

Those in private practice believe that nurses who work in agencies can grow only in limited ways, that they must play the bureaucratic games, that they must adapt to the medical model, and that they must focus on illness. Those supporting the agency model see it as the only model to provide comprehensive health care. They cite the need for many experts to provide the best primary care.

Some nurses in private practice say the practice of nursing does not require medical supervision, while those in agencies generally say that comprehensive care is not possible without delegation (with consequent supervision) of medical practice.

This issue will not be resolved soon. It is to be hoped that some of the emotionalism will subside so that the two models can be observed, described, documented, and studied. It would seem that each has something to offer a dynamic profession on the move.

SEX DISCRIMINATION IN HEALTH CARE POLICY

Despite the women's movement, affirmative-action legislation, and the emergence of politically active groups in nursing, there are very few women and fewer nurses involved in health care planning and policy-level activities. The chance of a private nurse practitioner being appointed to policy and planning boards is even more remote than the chances for nurses who work in agencies. Mayors, governors, and legislators, when looking for a token woman for a health care policy group, usually turn to deans of university schools of nursing or directors of nursing services. There is rarely more than one token woman. Unless nurse practitioners as a group become more active politically, their position will not be adequately represented in policymaking bodies, and the representation they do have will consist of nurses who are part of the existing system and who subscribe to it.

ISSUES NOT CONSIDERED

There are other critical issues that were not the focus of this conference but were often mentioned in passing. These included cost of comprehensive health care, distribution of health care services, professional nursing versus technical nursing and quality care, professional goals of nursing versus quality health care goals, fitting specialized nurse practitioners into the health care system versus fragmentation of health care services, continuing education and short-term education versus formal educational degree programs to prepare nurse practitioners, and ANA certification versus state licensure (or certification), or both, for nurse practitioners.

The most emotionally laden issue which was not considered at the conference relates to academic credentials of nurse practitioners. The majority of this group appears to have either diplomas or associate degrees in nursing. Preparation for expanded practice was largely in a 3- or 4-month university-sponsored intensive course followed by preceptorship training in a physician's office for a period of time ranging from several months to a year. A smaller group was prepared in a 2-year master's program. Those prepared at the master's level believe this is minimal preparation for nurse practitioners. Nursing would have a greater influence on health care legislation if the number of nurse practitioners holding the master's degree numbered in the thousands, rather than in the hundreds, which is the case. The writing of national health legislation cannot be greatly influenced by such a small group in any discipline, nor can they have widespread impact on health care. Compromises are slow in coming.

REFERENCES

1. Kissam PC: Physician's assistant and nurse practitioner: a study of health law reform. Kansas Law Review 24:1, 1975
2. Hall VC: Statutory Regulation of the Scope of Nursing Practice—A Critical Survey. Chicago, National Joint Practice Commission, 1975

CHAPTER 12

Charting the Course Ahead

With the radical and rapidly developing change brought by the nurse practitioner movement, all other components of the health care system experience pressure. There must be shifts in focus or function; readjustments and modifications are required. As with all changes in systems, communication of information speeds up and is subject to distortion. The threat of change brings resistance and creates new power alignments. The increasing complexities of society and the health care system also make any change more complex; change has many ramifications. It may become difficult for change agents (the nurse practitioners in this case) to plan and implement change, deal with resistance, and chart the course ahead. In addition to charting a course through a complex health world, nurse practitioners need to set priorities carefully.

INCREASED CLINICAL KNOWLEDGE AND EXPERTISE OF NURSES

To deliver effective, high-quality care to the people, nurses must obtain the best educational base possible, the best supervised practice, and the best continuing education or peer review. In responding to a question about what advice they would give to a nurse contemplating independent practice, almost all participants stressed knowledge and skill. Regardless of title, regardless of practice laws, the nurse practitioner movement will not be a viable component of the health care system without scholarship and clinical expertise. The wide distribution and isolation of nurse practitioners make this priority, or parts of it, difficult. Opportunities to meet in order to identify needs, criticize educational programs, and refine peer review processes should be provided and supported. These opportunities might be provided without taking a position of supporting or not supporting the movement, but rather to study the movement and the ways its problems are solved. A clearinghouse might be developed and supported for a period of time. This would provide a mechanism for directing people to educational programs they need, to people from whom they could receive certain kinds of clinical supervision, or to communities or health care groups that need someone with the nurse practitioner's particular skills. A clearinghouse might even provide consultation for nurse practitioners as they work out contracts with communities, physicians, and health care agencies or as they confront serious business, legal, political, or clinical problems in their practice. Again, support of a clearinghouse need not be with approval or disapproval of the movement, but rather another way of studying various aspects of the movement through active involvement in it.

DOING RESEARCH AT ALL LEVELS OF THE MOVEMENT

Most of the studies done up to this time are descriptive or reportorial in nature in terms of particular nurses, particular nurse practitioner programs, or graduates of particular programs. Some studies have documented that nurse practitioners are effective and productive, but data about cost and effect on patient welfare are limited.

There is a serious lack of research on the impact of nurse practitioners on the health care system, even in single communities. In the studies that have been done there are serious methodologic problems and problems in generalizing from particular to general groups. As part of the need for research on the impact of the nurse practitioner on the health care system, we need methodologies that permit more rigorous study.

We also need to look at community response, community acceptance of nurse practitioners, and factors within communities that influence how nurse practitioners are used and how effective their practices are. Research that documents health-promoting, growth-inducing functions, as well as advocacy and facilitative functions, needs to be done. Research that permits evaluation of quality as well as quantity of care provided by nurse practitioners is critical to the survival of the movement.

Lynn P. Dolins reports, "A large body of policy related research on human resources has been created over the last quarter century. However, its usefulness to decision-makers has been limited because it has not been evaluated comprehensively with respect to technical quality, usefulness to policymakers, and potential for codification and wider diffusion. In addition, this research has been hard to locate and is not easily accessible."[1] Nursing must align nurse practitioner research efforts in terms of political impact and usefulness, in addition to making it readily available to policymaking groups. There is little point in giving a high priority to research if it is not going to be accessible to those who need it most.

A nationwide survey completed by a panel of 341 nurses and non-nurses[2] probing priorities for clinical nursing research using the Delphi technique included 3 items related to nurse practitioners in the 15 items having the highest mean scores in terms of nursing taking the research leadership:[3]

Item 2: After clarifying the concept, evaluate the effects of expanding the role of the nurse in patient care.
Item 5: Delimit and evaluate the functions or clinical parameters of the independent nurse practitioners.
Item 9: Evaluate, in terms of patient outcomes, the role of the nurse in preventive health services.

The same 3 items ranked in the top 15 items when the total group of respondents rated items in terms of "value for the profession." They did not fall in the top 15 priorities (top 10 percent) when the panel rated items in terms of "impact on patient welfare." None of these items appeared in the top 10 percent when rated for "impact on patient welfare" when the respondents were separated into nurses and non-nurses or when they were divided into clinicians, administrators, educators, researchers, and "others." It appears that nurses and other respondents believe that nursing should take the leadership in studying the nurse practitioner because it would have value for the profession, not because of the potential of a great impact on patient welfare. This may reflect the urgent need for the profession to focus on patient welfare and have greater impact on the development of health care policy.

RESOLUTION OF MINORITY-GROUP ALIENATED BEHAVIOR

Nurses should give a high priority to resolving their own destructive behaviors. Pettiness, put-downs, backbiting, sabotaging, and drumming dissidents out of the profession have usually been blamed on the nature of interaction among women when they have to work with each other. But it is irrational to think that women are less loving, less supportive, less concerned than men or that men are required to keep women in line. Alienation theory helps us understand the rage, destructiveness, jealousy, envy, and intolerance of one nurse in relation to the growth or success of another. Our alienated behavior arises out of centuries of subjugation as women and more than 100 years of subjugation as nurses. Alienated people take on the values that are ascribed to them by those who subjugate them. If women are inferior to men and nurses are inferior to physicians, how can we allow women nurses to succeed, to become creative, to become activists, or to become important in the delivery of health care or the development of health care policy?

Nurses need to develop individual and group consciousness about how we keep our sister colleagues down, how we detract from and undermine their successes. We need to restructure our values and our behavior, hard as that may be, so that we encourage and foster advancement of our colleagues into positions of status, power, and prestige. The closer nurses move to where the decisions are made, the happier we should be. We need to be able to rejoice when members of the group earn degrees or become certified as nurse practitioners. We need to stop agreeing with physicians who say that nurses are overeducated or are trying to be junior doctors. We need to take issue when medicine envisions controlling our best practitioners as "physician extenders." What a put-down term! We need to recognize and accommodate a wide range of behaviors, recognizing that nurses who are militant, those who are political, those who manipulate, those who are expert in public relations all have roles to play if we can tap their particular talents. We must stop deploring when nurses "who do not know nursing" or "who don't have the right credentials" are put in positions of power. A detailed knowledge of nursing may not be important in terms of other talents people bring to a job. We need *to work* toward being truly glad and joyful at every woman's success, every nurse's success. Each promotion, each election, each accomplishment opens and expands the possibilities for every other member of the group.

Organized nursing needs to intervene in this ubiquitous and pernicious problem. In publications and meetings nurses could be made aware of alienated behaviors. Awareness groups and "Who Am I?" clinics could be included in meetings and even offered in continuing education programs. The pervasive low self-concept of nursing is only in the early stages of resolution. We need to provide a pattern of good ego trips for the members of our group.

NURSING ACCEPTANCE OF ALTERNATIVE MODELS OF PRACTICE

The name-calling and belittling of nurses who have departed from the medical model of practice and subscribed to the medical model of payment for services reflect the alienated behavior discussed above; this is professional self-destruction. Nursing's history of alienation certainly makes that one facet of the hostile dynamism set up when the nurses who subscribe to the demands of the emerging health care system meet with the nurses in private practice. "Self-serving," "narcissistic," "passé," "unfaithful to the people," "overserving the middle class," "junior doctor," "trying to be a big shot," "ignorant of health care needs" are epithets and accusations fired at practitioners. Private practitioners respond by calling their detractors "biased," "narrow-minded," "dogmatic," "armchair philosophers," who are "ignorant of what people really want in health care." They often note that those who derogate the loudest have never made a commitment to be accountable for a patient case load and, while sitting at a desk collecting $30,000 to $45,000 per year, do not know anything about either the financial risk or the risk to one's career that independent practice requires.

We need a moratorium on name-calling and a period of reserved judgment. We need a truce for awhile. We need to put monetary values on nursing services and to get acceptance for this value at local, state, and national levels. The nurse practitioners may just do it. We need to observe and support, if we can, the nurses who make a place in the community for dynamic health care practice. We have said that in the future 70 percent of the nurses will be working in the community. Are we going to chop off the heads of the first ones who go out there with something new to offer? If we finish them off, who will lead the way? We need to be able to listen as they describe what clients want and what they are doing. As nursing becomes more clearly defined as a practice, it may be because of this growing edge, this pushing into new frontiers. If we envy these nurses, but are not able to join them or emulate them, perhaps awareness of the envy will help to keep our minds open and our mouths shut. This is not to say that there are not critical questions that need to be raised. If the critical questions take the form of attack, counterattack will take the place of answers.

These nurses must be supported by their colleagues as they move out of the system and into uncharted territory. They must take their own responsibility for deviating from the system and for going against the tide. When they do plug into the system again, it may be that they will enrich health care and the profession.

CONCEPTUAL CHANGES IN NURSING PRACTICE ACTS

Hall[4] and Kissam[5] have done exhaustive surveys of the medical and nursing practice acts that have been changed to allow for expanded nursing functions. In addition, Kissam studied assistant physician legislation. Only a few states have made conceptual changes in their nursing practice acts. New York and California were the first, and some elements of the New York model have been incorporated into the definitions of nursing practice in several other states. The New York act defines nursing in conceptual terms and gets away from an activity-task definition. However, as noted previously, the New York act does not extend the scope of nursing practice beyond the traditional boundaries in the area of medicine. California, on the other hand, projects an increasing overlap of nursing and medical functions and recognition of nursing as a dynamic progressive discipline that will develop increasingly significant care activities. This statute permits interpretation of large areas of health care practice as belonging to both medicine and nursing.

Beyond these two conceptual concerns, nursing needs to search for ways to control nursing practice. Both joint boards and jointly prepared rules and regulations provide access for medical control and pressure. We are past the day when the nursing practice act can be considered alone. Any change in nursing requires adjustments at other levels, at least in medicine and possibly in other disciplines.

Careful planning of strategy and skill in negotiating are the requisites for any move to change nursing statutes.

GIVING DIRECTION TO HEALTH CARE

For a couple of decades we have had a great deal more knowledge about disease prevention and health promotion than we have been able to apply in the lives of people. Using fairly simple criteria we can project the major health risk for the next 5 years for almost anyone. Medicine, generally, is not interested in health, and the bureaucracy most nurses work in does not value either disease prevention or health promotion. The major techniques used in the past have been exhortation and, failing that, inducing fear in the client. We have given little attention to client goals; thus we know little about how disease prevention, health promotion, or human growth activities conflict with these goals. We know few motivating strategies, few strategies for working through conflicting goals and needs, and few techniques for placing responsibility on the client. Facilitation strategies, for the most part, are still to be worked out. Independent nurse practitioners are in a unique position to develop and test a discipline of health care. They are making a beginning in identifying and supporting health in their clients.

Teaching techniques related to health care are still in their infancy. Teaching problem-solving techniques to individuals and groups may be critical to health care. For example, just dealing with the problems of whether to take the pill, whether to have an abortion, whether to have a vasectomy, or whether to have a baby after the age of 40 years requires high levels of problem-solving and teaching skills. One could list critical choices with which clients might need assistance for every specialty.

Advocacy as a nursing role is still virgin territory. With the increasing complexity in scientific technology and the health care system, as well as the increasing numbers of alternatives in health care, advocacy may well be a major facilitative role for nurses. There is still little documentation for the role, but one can begin to visualize its helpfulness to clients.

Closely allied to health promotion is the function of active support of growth processes. In the past, nursing, like medicine, looked for failures in growth and for immaturities. Nurses have done little to support mothering and fathering and have provided little affirmation of growth in health or illness. This is another area in which the frontiers of nursing could be advanced.

Counseling in minor and major life crises also seems to be an evolving role for nurses. Helping people solve such problems as an impasse in wedding plans, helping mothers separate from children when they become of school age, providing rape crisis care and follow-up counseling, and counseling the incest victim and sex offender are all areas nurses are entering. There is still little literature on counseling a large ambulatory population. No other group of health workers is in a better position to develop and document the discipline of health care.

MECHANISMS FOR COMMUNICATION

Participants at the conference almost unanimously expressed a need for communication with each other and with other nurse practitioners in independent and private practice. A wide variety of reasons for meeting were given, without any central focus. Beyond the personal reasons of affirmation, self-validation, and support, it would seem that documentation of practice, business procedures, success with third-party payers, and solutions to practice, political, legal, and business problems, as well as examination of published research, would be valid reasons for meeting. Work sessions concerning practice might provide input from the group to the profession at large. Organized nursing might provide input to the practitioner group about developments in health policy. The survival of the nurse practitioner movement may be related to developing mechanisms for communication within the group and between the group and the profession. Survival may also be related to how dynamic the communication is and how well it meets the needs of the group.

REFERENCES

1. Cohen Ed, et al (eds): An Evaluation of Policy Related Research on New and Expanded Roles of Health Workers. New Haven, Yale University School of Medicine, 1974, p v
2. Lindeman CA: Delphi Survey of Clinical Nursing Research Priorities. Boulder, Colo, Western Interstate Commission for Higher Education, 1974, p 9

3. Ibid, p 23
4. Hall VC: Statutory Regulation of the Scope of Nursing Practice—A Critical Survey. Chicago, National Joint Practice Commission, 1975
5. Kissam PC: Physician's assistant and nurse practitioner laws: a study in health law reform. Kansas Law Review 24:1, 1975

SECTION III

APPENDICES

APPENDIX A

The University of Iowa College of Nursing

Organization for the Practice of Psychiatric Nursing
National Invitational Conference, December 11–12, 1975

Supported by
The National Institute of Mental Health

Final Program

December 11

8:30 A.M.	Registration, coffee and rolls; Michigan Room
9:00	Welcome; Evelyn R. Barritt, Dean, College of Nursing, University of Iowa
9:15	Introductions and Conference Plans; Ada Jacox, Project Codirector
9:30	How Come; Why Now?—The Nurse Practitioner Movement; Catherine Norris, Project Codirector
10:00	Perspectives on Professional Practice; Loretta Ford, Dean, University of Rochester School of Nursing
10:45	Coffee

11:00 Response of Conference Group; Response Leader, Elizabeth Carter, Chairperson, Interim Executive Committee, Council of Advanced Practitioners in Psychiatric Mental Health Nursing, American Nurses' Association

12:00 Lunch

1:00 P.M. Small Group Work: Each participant will have signed up in the morning for two small groups for afternoon work. Group limits are 7–10 members.

- Group 1: The Law–Issues and Problems; Leader, Janelle Ramsburg; Michigan Room
- Group 2: Economics and Malpractice Insurance; Leader, Madeleine Gerrish; Harvard Room
- Group 3: Identification of Health Needs, Clientele, and Scope of Services; Leader, Josephine Van der Meer; Princeton Room
- Group 4: Preparation for Independent Nursing Practice including Standards of Certification; Leader, Ingeborg Mauksch; Northwestern Room
- Group 5: Policy Development–Kinds and Areas of Policy; Leader, Gertrude Isaacs; Hoover Room
- Group 6: Strategies for Selling Services to Others, Clients, and Professionals; Leader, Evelyn Barritt; Grant Wood Room

3:00 Coffee

3:20

- Group A: Strategies for Selling Services to Others, Clients, and Professionals: Leader, Patty Brandner; Michigan Room
- Group B: Evaluation and Research of Services and Effectiveness of Nurses; Leader, Carolyn Williams; Harvard Room
- Group C: Fee Schedule and Third-Party Payments; Leader, Karlene Kerfoot; Princeton Room
- Group D: Identification of Health Needs, Clients, and Scope of Services; Leader, Sarah Archer; Northwestern Room
- Group E: Forms of Association with Other Professionals; Leader, Sharon Gedan; Hoover Room
- Group F: Loose Thinkers and Dreamers; Leader, Lorene Fisher; Grant Wood Room

December 12

8:15 Coffee and rolls

8:30 Scope of Practice: Inclusions and Exclusions; On Whom Should You Rely? Marvin Fish

9:00 Discussion by Large Group; Discussion Leader, Helen Grace

9:30 The Nursing Business: Take Two Aspirin and Call Me in the Morning; Lawrence Subrin

10:00 Open Discussion

10:30 Coffee

11:00 Four Small Group Discussions: Legal Implications or Economic Aspects of Independent and Private Nursing Practice; groups on legal implications, Marvin Fish, resource person; groups on economic implications, Lawrence Subrin, resource person

Legal 1: Leader, Nancy Tally; Princeton Room

Legal 2: Leader, Karlene Kerfoot; Purdue Room

Economics 1: Leader, Lucille Kinlein; Minnesota Room

Economics 2: Leader, Margaret Wacker; Michigan Room

12:30 Lunch

1:30 Two Group Meetings:

Group A: Developing a Mechanism for Private Practitioners Communicating with Each Other; Leader, Nancy Keller; Michigan Room

Group B: Communication Needs and Mechanisms for Independent Nursing Practitioners; Where do we go from here? Do we need other kinds of projects? Leader, Karlene Kerfoot; Princeton Room

2:30 Summary; Loretta Ford and Evelyn Barritt

Highlights of Conference

Priorities for the Profession

Viability and Health of the Nurse Practitioner Movement—Private Nursing Practice Movement

Observations or remarks of official representatives: NIMH Division of Nursing, ANA, and resource people

Closure; Ada Jacox, Catherine Norris

APPENDIX B

Profile of Participants

Our purpose in developing a profile of practice was to determine the range and variation of organization, practices, clientele, policies, and problems within the nurse practitioner movement. At this point in our development it may be more useful to look at the possibilities and examine the range than to look at a group profile or a mean or to try to categorize or classify too rigidly. Thus many direct quotations are presented to give the flavor of the responses, rather than providing a simple count.

Item 21. The critical incidents were too numerous to do more than exemplify each category of incident (see Chapter 8). This summary represents 37 participants who completed the participant profile questionnaire.

COMPILATION OF PARTICIPANT PROFILE SHEETS

1. Names and addresses (see chapter 1).
2. Location of practice

West (13 states)	13
Midwest (12 states)	11
South (16 states)	7
East (9 states)	6

3. Name of practice or agency

	Nursing Dynamics Corporation	
	Counseling Associates	
	Frontier Nursing Service	
	Nursing Consultation	
	Community Nurse Practitioners	
	Nursing Care and Consultation, Ltd.	
	Alternatives in Health Care	
	Visiting Nurse Service (one-nurse private practice)	
	Health Care Associates	
	Neurosurgical Associates, P.A.	
	Iowa Veterans Home	
	Northwest Family Health Center	
	School of Medicine, Family Care Center	
	Creative Health Services	
	Kaiser–Permanente Medical Group	
	Expansion Inc.	
	Med-Air Corporation	
	County Mental Health Service	
	Family Nursing Care	
	Employee in practice with a physician	
	Private practice, individual name	9
	Faculty of college	3
	No answer	1
4.	Income	
	Full-time profit	21
	Full-time nonprofit	12
	Part-time nonprofit	5
	Part-time profit	3
5a.	Formal organization for practice	
	Individual practice	14
	H.C. agency or college-employed	9
	Corporation	7
	Partnership	2
	Private group	2
	Individual practice and partnership	1
	Employee of physician	1
	No answer	1
5b.	Disciplines with which nurses practice	
	Medicine	24
	Nursing	9
	No answer	6
	Nutrition	4

	Women's health professional group	3
	Pharmacology	3
	Psychology	3
	Social work	3
	Self only	3
	Law	2
	Community mental health	1
	Sociology	1
	Biology	1
	HMO staff	1
	Hospital staff	1
	Adult education	1
	Public health	1
	Anthropology	1
	Economics	1
	Research	1
	Recreation	1
	Physical therapy	1
6a.	Scope of practice	
	Individual counseling or therapy	17
	Family counseling or therapy	13
	Group counseling or therapy	12
	Crisis intervention	8
	Teaching or training workshop	6
	Primary care	6
	Screening assessment and evaluation	6
	Patient teaching or instruction	5
	Consultation	4
	Health care program development	4
	Research	3
	No practice data given	3
	Staff-development and evaluation	2
	School health	2
	Couples therapy	2
	Supervision and management (clients)	2
	Cotherapist with physician	1
	Proposal formulation	1
	Publication	1
	Delegated medical care	1
6b.	Areas of practice	
	Mental health or psychiatric nursing	12
	Health education, care, and counseling	12

Physical illness, physical problems	10
Sex education and sexuality	6
Nursing techniques and care	6
Child psychology	3
Growth and development	3
Consciousness raising, awareness training	3
No practice data	3
Life style alteration	2
Community health	2
Medicolegal problems	1
Midwifery	1
Family, except obstetric services	1
Family practice	1

7a. Clients, number

Lack of precision in the question and lack of conformity in answering for this aspect of practice provided some interesting results. Some respondents identified the size of the population served; some identified the length of time they had been in practice and the total number of patients cared for in that time; others identified their weekly case load, and others their current case load.

Weekly case load:

75–150	4
10–20	2
50–75	2
35	1
6 individuals	1
12 groups	1
20–30	1
5–6 families	1
300 (corporation)	1
200	1

Monthly case load:

20–30 families	2
1 group	1
4 referrals	1

Total current case load:

40	1
80	1
36	1
10 + 3–5 waiting list	1
5 families, 15 individuals	1

Total load since going into practice:

125–130 in 2 years	1
200 in 3 years	1
6 in 3 months	1
No data given	11

7b. Clients

Health problems:
Long-term and chronic
Acute
Minor injuries/trauma
Child-rearing
Crisis
Character disorders/psychosocial dysfunction
Relationship
Emotional
Pre-op preparation
Complete range
Medication
Obstetrics and gynecology
Sex problems, offenders, victims
Nursing care need
Education and self-help
Assessment and evaluation
Geriatric/psychosocial
Growth and development
Health promotion
Disease prevention
Staff teaching
Medicolegal
Consultation on program, grant proposals, malpractice, research
Collaboration with other health professionals

7c. Clients, age

Complete range	14
Middle age	10
Geriatric	7
No data	6
Young adults	6
Children	3

7d. Clients, sex

Both	17
No data	8
Mostly women	6

	Male 40%, female 60%	4
	Male 10%, female 90%	1
	Mostly men	1
7e.	Clients, socioeconomic status	
	Middle	17
	All	10
	Lower	7
	Lower middle	6
	Upper	6
	No data	4
	Minority	1
7f.	Clients, rural–urban (number of times mentioned—some respondents listed all three)	
	Urban	25
	Rural	12
	Suburban	3
	No data	4
8.	Legal consultation	
	Yes	17
	No	17
	No answer	3
9.	CPA or economic consultation	
	Yes	16
	No	18
	No answer	3
10.	Advisory board	
	Yes	11
	No	21
	No answer	4
11.	Policy manual	
	Yes	12
	No	22
	No answer	2
12.	Medical backup	
	Yes	25
	No	6
	No answer	1
	Joint practice with medicine	3
	No answer	2
	Medical referral only	1
13.	Publicity materials	
	Yes	17

	No	18
	No answer	2
	Professional cards	
	Brochures	
	Posters	
	Letterheads on bills	
	Newspaper articles	
	Advertisements	
	Newsletters	
	Books	
	Articles in professional literature	
14.	Fee schedule	
	Yes	12
	No	20
	No answer	5
15.	Third-party payments	
	Yes	15
	No	17
	No answer	5
16.	Malpractice insurance	
	Yes	29
	No	3
	No answer	4

Where:	Amount:
ANA	Max 3,000,000; no amount given
CNA	250,000–500,000
Royal Globe	1,000,000–3,000,000
Continental	250,000 (200,000 personal, 600,000 professional)
Britton Agency, New Jersey	No amount given
St. Paul Fire & Marine	100,000–300,000
McGinnis & Associates, Chicago	No amount given
Cannot divulge name of company	No amount given
"My own"	No amount given
In process, Kaiser–Permanente Policy	No amount given
Through hospital carrier	No amount given

One respondent took the position that she was "not really coverable" since she was working beyond the "usual scope of practice outside of an established medical facility—in a senior center and in the community."

17.	Broad areas of greatest problems	
	Economics and business	4

Learning the world of business	1
Getting paid for my expertise in the health field	1
Following up and collecting fees	1
Fees are a barrier to utilization of services	1
Naiveté about business practices	1
Hesitancy about discussing fees with patients	1
I like what I'm doing so well that I give it away free	1
Bookkeeping	1
Procuring knowledge of funding sources	1
Getting good business advice	1
Would like to establish fee standards	1
Making decisions about business practices and insurance problems	1
Lack of information about how to go about it	1
Economic considerations in relation to client's private physician	1
Total, economics and business	18
Lack of knowledge among professionals about professional nursing:	
I have to explain my contributions in health promotion to the M.D.	2
I needed to explain my skills to a psychiatrist	1
Psychiatrists know that social workers are private therapists, but not that psychiatric nurses are	1
We have spent a lot of time convincing colleagues through words and actions that people need and will use our services	1
There is simply unawareness of nurse therapists in private practice	1
It took awhile to educate a few doctors	1
Educating nurses as well as other disciplines that psychiatric nursing clinical specialists are capable of quality therapy	1
Inexperience of judges in accepting nurse expert witness	1
Probably the most difficult area has been receiving recognition (with commensurate pay) for my expertise in the health field	1
Physician acceptance	1
Isolated threats by physicians in state to nurses doing preventive, primary, and health care maintenance	1
Total, lack of knowledge	12

Getting recognition for third-party payments	9
We are preparing our baseline data for presentation to third-party payers	1
Third-party payment is the usual way most people pay for health services, and these do not pay for a self-employed nurse therapist	1
Acceptance (lack of it) by third-party payer	1
Total, third-party payment problems	12
Generating clientele	2
I had to compete with psychiatrists (residents) for patients referred for psychotherapy; I found nurses often got the severest problems	1
Getting referrals from physicians	1
Developing referral sources or base	1
Must find clients, so am forced to do some public relations	1
Establishing myself in a field no other nurses were involved in	1
Being referred appropriate clients and not just those who require physical care	1
Setting limits on numbers and kinds of patients (resulted in exhaustion)	1
Assessing attorneys who wish to avail themselves of my services	1
Lack of communication from physicians in the immediate area of practice	1
Total, generating clientele	11
Negativism and lack of support from nurses	2
Peer awareness and acceptance (other R.N.'s)	2
No referrals from nurses	1
Other nurses wish to control all nurses' in-house activities	1
The most serious problem I see is that of convincing nurses that nursing care is needed after hospital discharge	1
Total, nurse negativism	7
Legal problems	1
Licensure for practice	1
The gray–black area that restricts nurses from practicing alone; only when I decided to risk whatever in order to share my skills with the public was I able to take a chance	1

One hospital administration is questioning the legality of my position	1
That of comfort with pioneering role before there is legal backup	1
Considering and deciding about legalities of practice	1
Lack of legal base	1
Total, legal problems	7
Developing own convictions about role and therapy	
Role realignment	1
Breaking out of the dependent practitioner model	1
I had to synthesize many theoretical frameworks and develop my own convictions about treatment	1
Total, developing own conviction about practice	3
Personal	
Boredom: I was just seeing 1- to 3-year-olds for well checks	
Patience: I prefer practice to public relations; I don't like to take time to sell myself	1
We have been providing services on a voluntary basis or donations consistently since February 1974; now it's beginning to pay off; we have proven both value and need	1
Knowledge: I needed to expand my knowledge of assessment of all patient problems	1
Fear of failure	1
Fear of a lawsuit	1
Fear of public disapproval	1
Fear of agency administration disapproval	1
Total, personal problems	8
Interpreting professional nursing to consumers	1
Educating consumers that nursing has some valuable services to offer and that health care is not the same as illness care	2
There is difficulty getting across to patients that doctors want them to receive care, that nursing is not a competitive field; they fear abandonment by the doctor if he doesn't order nursing	1
About half the public thought I was only caring for the poor	1
Consumers are just not aware of nursing	1
Unlearning some things about nursing (nurse–patient relationships) from clients' point of view	1

Combating community consumer orientation to crisis health care delivery	1
Low level of health education	1
Total, interpretation to consumers	9
Miscellaneous	
Getting hospital privileges	2
Cultural: male-dominated society, including most nurses, do not think we can work without some "big daddy" telling us what to do	1
Support: getting more than individual (nonfinancial) support from local community leaders	1
Resources: commanding resources to serve a volume of clients	1
Keeping the group of practitioners together	1
Finding a physician to work with	1
Difficulty in getting patients to specialized referral services due to distances, lack of transportation, money	1
Local community politics	1
Total, miscellaneous problems	9
No answer	1
Not applicable	1

APPENDIX C

Descriptions of Practice

A FAMILY PSYCHOTHERAPY PRACTICE

Margaret Wacker

I began my private practice in psychiatric nursing when I decided that I wanted to do good family psychotherapy and discovered how very difficult it was for a nurse to do this in traditional health care settings. My total initial investment included an answering-service machine and a minimal amount of printed materials, which included business cards and stationery. I was able to reduce costs by using a room in my home as an office. I purchased ANA malpractice insurance at a cost of $15 per year. My practice built slowly but steadily. During the first year I had to devote a great deal of time to promoting myself as a capable family psychotherapist. My most productive referral base came out of my contacting mental health agencies in the community and requesting a multicrisis family unable to afford private therapy. I agreed to see them without cost as a community service. Once I was interviewed and presented my credentials, I was assigned a family. I used this opportunity as a model for the clinic, where they could view what I was able to accomplish and thereby develop their own assessment of my clinical ability. Since the family was known in great detail to most of the staff, it was easy for them to follow the progress. A clinical nurse specialist became more than a fancy title that no one really understood. It became a reality, a person they liked and whose clinical abilities they were beginning to respect.

My theoretical underpinnings include Bowen theory[1] and Rogers' view[2] of synergistic man. It is my own synthesis of these theories that provides me with a positive view of the human condition in a universe of open systems. This positive view enables me to work with difficult family issues such as child abuse, divorce, and severe mental dysfunction. I find the medical model atavistic and hard to transcend. An open-system model encourages growth in all the family membership. It conveys many positive values, including hope.

I treat families in a variety of settings. I use my office about 50 percent of the time. The rest of the time I see families in their homes or in school settings. At home I find family process more palpable than in my office. Somehow people are more like themselves when relating from the context in which they live.

School visits are always productive. I find that my efforts to neutralize the reactions between teacher and child place difficult school behavior into an understandable framework. This gets the teacher out of cause-and-effect thinking. If she believes that a child is just lazy, she will engage in behavior directed toward getting at his laziness. If she understands the key family process operating on the child, her interventions can be more relevant to his specific needs.

Presenting problems, the sine qua non of the medical model focus, disappear as foci when their roots are traced to family process. This is particularly true when the presenting problem is a labeled patient. I convey as early as possible in my work with the family that I don't see the child as sick. I see instead an unhealthy family process. The child is just making it easy for everyone to avoid working on their part in it. The usual response is an increased effort to document the sickness in the child. This gives me additional clues. It is important for me to know which members have a need for a labeled patient. I have never found it possible to unlabel a patient without unhitching the process in the labeler as well.

The following case study illustrates my work with a particular multicrisis family:

The S. family was referred to me from the mental hygiene clinic in my town. The S. family consisted of one child from the present marriage, two from her previous marriage, and four from his previous marriage. The school that all seven children attended was embroiled in an intense negative process with the family. In their efforts to help, they had had psychologic testing done on five of the children, and they had diagnostic labels justifying a pressing need for immediate psychotherapy for all. The family and school were busy shouting at each other over issues such as "the family's neglecting to care for the children properly" and "the school's failure to teach the children."

My first operational principle was to relate to the family and the school without getting hooked into the feelings on either side. The principle of the Bowen triangle in families operates in systems outside the family also. I scheduled a meeting with every teacher involved with each child, as well as the school psychologist, nurse, and principal. My school contact centered on getting everyone to think about these children without reacting to them. I drew a family diagram and encouraged everyone to look at it as they presented their exasperated complaints. I broke into the reporting when feelings got intense with such comments as these: Did you know that Mary has the same name as Mr. S.'s first wife and John has the same name as Mrs. S.'s first husband? I wonder what that means in this family?

In addition, I gave the school personnel my home and office telephone numbers with instructions that they should feel free to call me regarding anything of importance concerning the S. family. I used the telephone medium to relate to all the most anxious people while at the same time staying out of the process. I constantly shaped the content of their calls with a more thoughtful look at the issues. For example: a teacher called regarding Mrs. S.'s refusal to allow Tom S. to spend a day on a farm with the rest of the class. She spent a great deal of time explaining that Tom needed this more than his classmates and that she could no longer tolerate Mrs. S.'s neglect of this child. I summarized the call with the thought that I wondered why Mrs. S. did not value this educational experience for her child. As it turned out, the teacher had presented the day to Mrs. S. as an effort to give him special attention and had failed to stress that this was an important educational experience for all children. When she was able to communicate this to Mrs. S. on the following day, Tom was allowed to attend.

I also spent a 30-minute observation period in each child's classroom for the purpose of making my own judgment about his in-school functioning. This observation period gave me the opportunity to collect important data for later use. Gradually the stress began to get toned down between these two systems. During a session with the family and another at the school, I drew a diagram of what I thought was happening between them:

Constant exasperated complaints by the school to the family.

↓

Mrs. S. felt they were putting her down as a mother.

↓

Mrs. S. put the school down, criticized, and resisted cooperating with them.

This diagram and explanation enabled the members of each system to think about what was going on between them. Within 1 month the multiple telephone calls from school personnel and Mrs. S. decreased significantly. With this under control, I was able to bring up in the sessions with the S. family important issues concerning the children that both the family and the school seemed too uptight to see or to deal with. This included the battering of Ellen and the differential treatment of the children. The battering of Ellen grew out of Mrs. S.'s inability to discipline the children. She felt that since she was not the natural mother of the older S. children she could not discipline them. Since she could not discipline them, she could not justify disciplining her own J. children. When the children got out of control she looked the other way, and Ellen (the usual troublemaker) got beaten up by the older children. This changed when Mr. S. said that he expected her to discipline all the children and was getting damned tired of having to deal with her unfinished parental business when he came home from work each night. She began to take a stand with the kids, and with his support the children came under much better control.

The differential treatment of the children grew out of unstated feelings of resentment that each parent felt about having to take on the responsibilities for the other's children. Mr. S. said he resented having to support her two boys, but did it since she was taking care of his four. She said she hated having to take care of his four, but did it because he was supporting her two. As the parents began to work on improving their own functioning, the "his," "hers," and "our" camps broke up. This was actualized by the J. boys remaining in school for lunch each day, as the S. children always had, thus breaking up a highly resented pattern of a special lunchtime with their mother for the J. boys. In addition, the older S. children were no longer sent off to a day-care mother for 4 hours after school each day while the J. children went directly home.

By the tenth session we were talking about differentiation of each adult self. Mrs. S. had begun taking driving lessons and was looking for part-time employment. Mr. S. had worked so much overtime that he was no longer eligible for public assistance.

In conclusion, I would like to say that therapy is only as good as the theoretical framework and underlying philosophy from which it derives. When the philosophy is positive, working with strengths and underplaying the negative parts of the equation, even the multicrisis family gets a chance to catch its breath and grow.

REFERENCES

1. Bowen M: The use of family theory in clinical practice. Compr Psychiatry 7:345, 1966
2. Rogers M: Theoretical Basis of Nursing. Philadelphia, Davis, 1970

A FAMILY NURSE CLINICIAN IN A RURAL SETTING*

Carolyn V. Whitaker

Concern with the existing health care crisis and my dissatisfaction with the health care delivery system motivated me to go to graduate school. I hoped to be able to demonstrate better utilization of professional nurses in combating existing health care crises and ultimately to make a more satisfying career for myself. The graduate program for family nurse clinicans at Vanderbilt University is a 12-month program jointly sponsored by the schools of nursing and medicine. Nurses completing the program have clinical expertise in promoting wellness and preventing illness, in assessing health of families and individuals, in managing common deviations from health, and in providing maintenance care for stabilized patients with chronic health problems. Family nurse clinicians func-

**Revised from a paper presented before the National League for Nursing convention in 1975 at an open forum on maldistribution of health manpower, New Orleans, Louisiana, May 20, 1975. Published with permission of PSF Productions Corporation, Austin, Texas*

tion interdependently with other health professionals and refer patients for other health services when appropriate.

When I completed graduate study there was no organized plan of primary care delivery in Tennessee. So I had to create my own role in either a new or existing system. The task of beginning work was more difficult than my total graduate school experience. First I established guidelines for locating a setting for practice. They were (1) finding a place where I was wanted and needed, (2) having freedom to demonstrate the family nurse clinician role, (3) finding feasible financing for my service, (4) finding suitable linkage to other health care team members, and (5) locating a rural setting, by choice as well as to fulfill a commitment made as a condition of assistance while a graduate student.

A small town in Macon County, Tennessee, had been without health care for 15 years. The people in the community were articulate in identifying their health needs and were committed to seeking viable solutions. They expected to share in the planning, development, and implementation of a health service to meet those needs. At a town meeting I interpreted the role of a family nurse clinician. It was an exciting experience for me to work with such a highly motivated group. They posed many difficult questions based on very real and practical health problems they had had to face and solve. Community support grew in the form of petitions for the development of a family nurse clinic. A council was formed with charter and bylaws. Together we developed my contract with the council, organizational plans (both manpower and administrative), and financing of the clinical services.

We established a totally new subsystem of health care within the existing system. The newness of the role of family nurse clinician for a nurse made it imperative for me to seek counsel and guidance from established health care sources. Physicians inside and outside the proposed service area were consulted for referral and informational purposes. The county health department was consulted about collaborative relationships. The Tennessee Board of Pharmacy was consulted for guidance in planning safe and efficient use of pharmaceuticals. The Tennessee Nurses' Association and Tennessee Board of Nursing were asked to review our proposal. I obtained personal medical-legal assistance in developing the contractural agreement. The regional health planning council was involved from the first and served as counsel to the executive committee of our health care service. Tennessee Midsouth Regional Medical Program gave developmental assistance and provided financial support to demonstrate the role of the family nurse clinician. Funding for the first 8 months of operation totaled $24,000, of which about one-third was raised by the community. This support was used for lease of a building, renovation, equipment, supplies, salaries for staff, and other operating expenses.

The Family Nurse Service Clinic was a primary and maintenance health care service. In addition to me, the staff consisted of a clinic assistant. The clinic had three examining rooms, a laboratory, a drug room, a reception room, a records room, a teaching conference room, and an office for me. The assistant's responsibilities included office management, records, simple laboratory procedures, and assistance to the family nurse clinician. The family record system was based on a modified problem-oriented approach.

Health care services were delivered as I had conceptualized in my plan while a graduate student in the FNC program at Vanderbilt University.

My linkage with physicians was through a protocol that was given to all physicians in the surrounding area. The protocol contained a pharmaceutical formulary used in managing over 100 common deviations from wellness once I made the diagnosis.

One physician in the area served, by letter of commitment, as sponsoring physician. This collaborative sponsorship was on a volunteer basis. I contacted my sponsor at least every week. He was available for consultation at any time, despite the fact that his office was located 18 miles away. Interaction with physicians was determined by patient preference. A patient who did not have a physician but who needed one was referred using a rotating monthly schedule of physicians. Patients I saw were required to provide me with the names of their personal physicians. Prescriptions for drugs were cosigned by family nurse clinician and physician. I was available in the clinic 5½ days or 43 hours weekly. I scheduled home visits for mornings and afternoons. Emergencies in the clinic and home were handled as they occurred.

I sponsored a community health education program, responding to the community's choice of a weight-reduction program. The group held weekly meetings. After meeting weekly for 6 months the 63 members in the group had achieved a total weight loss of 650 pounds.

Residents of the area serviced by the clinic became actively involved through a volunteer program. Over 600 hours of volunteer time were provided in 6 months. Volunteers interested in exploring health careers spent afternoons, Saturdays, and weekdays during the summer assisting in the clinic.

The patients using the service were articulate in stating what they wanted out of their clinic visits, even to the extent of telling me they wanted "a shot of penicillin for a cold." It might be said that the community was a "shot"-oriented group. Because of transportation problems, emergency rooms in the area hospitals were frequently used for primary illnesses. Often patients received "shots" for their complaints and were told to go to see their physicians the next day. People were accustomed to this type of health care. It was frustrating to me to try to provide quality health care while having to meet expectations of the consumers for care. This fee-for-service clinic had an increased impact on me because I had never had such contractual agreements with consumers.

In assessing community health care needs, I found the greatest need was health education. Until such education could be provided, I would continue to have conflicts about delivery of health care. The notion of a "shot" to get the patient better was deep-rooted in several generations of the community. I had to cope with this until patients understood how medications were absorbed in the body and how they helped in illness.

Miller et al[1] studied the clinic's utilization during its first 7 months of operation. I kept comprehensive records of various demographics, chief complaints, tests performed, treatments, dispositions, and payments. Time waited and time seen were kept for each patient seen by the family nurse clinician. The clinic assistant kept a daily log that included 13 categories including patient's age, name, and sex, old or new patient, clinic or home visit, nature of complaint, tests performed, and therapy prescribed. Additional data included patient disposition, whether a return appointment was requested, and length of the visit to the clinic.

This descriptive study of patient utilization of a family nurse clinician shows the extent to which a specially trained master's-level nurse can function as a relatively independent practitioner in a rural area. During the 7-month period a total of 1407 patients made 1781 visits to the clinic. Family registration totaled 643 families. I diagnosed and provided care for patients with problems ranging from lacerations, burns, sore throats, and flu to broken bones, urinary infections, diabetes, arthritis, and heart attacks. Other problems included enuresis and emotional problems related to school and family relationships, in addition to problems of families and individuals learning to cope with chronic illness, terminal illness, and aging. Most patients received a physical examination (either partial or complete), all but 14 percent of the patients had one or more tests, and drugs or prescriptions for drugs were distributed to 61 percent of the patients.

I referred only 140 of the 1781 patients I saw. More than 70 percent of the referrals were to physicians, while the majority of the others were to health agencies. This finding suggests that a family nurse clinician in a rural area can expect that the majority of the conditions presented to her will not require outside consultation. It is not known, however, whether the distribution of complaints brought to my attention were self-selective (ie, persons with symptoms of a more acute nature went directly to a physician or other source) or whether this distribution represented a full constellation of health problems in the clinic catchment area.

The substantial increase in repeat patient utilization of the clinic over the 7-month period indicates that the clinic might be able to meet operating expenses without outside funding. Repeat patient utilization is also suggestive of patient satisfaction.

Return visits and increased utilization of maintenance care can be attributed to the development of a patient–family nurse clinician trust relationship, the convenience of the health services, and the relatively low cost of the care provided.

Our budget limited the number and type of laboratory tests available. More equipment for conducting laboratory tests would have permitted better service. However, additional staff would have been required.

The unique arrangement of an independent family nurse clinician contracting with a local nonprofit community group to provide primary and maintenance health care allowed the service area residents to continue their choice of physician linkage, while at the same time having a point of entry into the health field in their community.

The data in this study indicate that a family nurse clinician can provide economical primary and maintenance health care to deprived areas of our society.

Much education of physicians and nurses was required continuously. News media such as television and newspapers were utilized in the forms of feature and news stories; I participated in documentary films and spoke to professional nursing and medical society meetings. I spent many personal hours meeting these commitments. Some of these occasions were controversial. It has required a great deal of personal leadership in demonstrating nursing's competence for assuming more responsibility and accountability for decision-making in an evolving health care delivery system.

All that begins well does not always end well. There were problems. The community's notion of the health care they needed was based on the model they knew 20 to 30 years ago. Solo practice was not and is not conducive to good health for consumer or provider.

The starvation of a community for health care produced possessive behavior in clients that caused barriers in communication and made my life miserable. There were few opportunities for me to have continuing education experiences. There came a time when trade-offs in negotiations between provider and consumer were exhausted. A small group of the board of directors became impatient. A group of physicians in an adjoining county overextended their economical ratio of physician provider to consumer and became interested in staffing the clinic. The question arose whether the clinic could support my services and those of the physician group. The board opted to reorganize the service using physicians on a basis of 5 days per week for 6 hours daily. No home visit service was available even in emergency, and none of the physicians providing the service would live in the community. This reorganization lasted 8 months. Then the clinic doors closed permanently. Many persons say it was due to lack of community support. The physicians said they were forced to close because a physician left the group and they were unable to provide adequate service.

From the first day I opened the clinic people in the community seemed to need my continuous reassurance that I would not leave. I have not left the community, even though I am in joint practice with a physician approximately 20 miles away. I continue to see many of my clinic families. As I move about the community I am often asked not to move away: "We feel so much better because you are here. We don't know what we would do without you. This town will never get a doctor. What we need is a nurse. The Family Nurse Service Clinic should never have closed." My telephone continues to ring in the early morning and evening hours with the ever familiar remark, "Carolyn, please tell me what I should do. . . ." I continue to be the health provider–counselor for this deprived area.

I do not advocate solo-provider health care delivery. Health team linkage is a must. Health care cannot be provided by one individual alone. Primary health care is and should be a 24-hour/day 7-day/week service. This requires a multidiscipline team of people, in addition to a well-developed referral system.

REFERENCE

1. Miller MH, Whitaker CV, Dennis C, George V, Reynolds WJ: Utilization of a Family Nurse Service Clinic. Vanderbilt University, Nashville, Tenn. Unpublished presentation to American Public Health Association annual meeting, San Francisco, Calif, November 1973

Index